Embodiment and everyday cyborgs

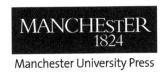

Manchester University Press

INSCRIPTIONS

Series editors
Des Fitzgerald and Amy Hinterberger

Editorial advisory board
Vivette García Deister, National Autonomous University of Mexico
John Gardner, Monash University, Australia
Maja Horst, Technical University of Denmark
Robert Kirk, Manchester, UK
Stéphanie Loyd, Laval University, Canada
Alice Mah, Warwick University, UK
Deboleena Roy, Emory University, USA
Hallam Stevens, Nanyang Technological University, Singapore
Niki Vermeulen, Edinburgh, UK
Megan Warin, Adelaide University, Australia
Malte Ziewitz, Cornell University, USA

Since the very earliest studies of scientific communities, we have known that texts and worlds are bound together. One of the most important ways to stabilise, organise and grow a laboratory, a group of scholars, even an entire intellectual community, is to write things down.
As for science, so for the social studies of science: Inscriptions is a space for writing, recording and inscribing the most exciting current work in sociological and anthropological – and any related – studies of science.
The series foregrounds theoretically innovative and empirically rich interdisciplinary work that is emerging in the UK and internationally. It is self-consciously hospitable in terms of its approach to discipline (all areas of social sciences are considered), topic (we are interested in all scientific objects, including biomedical objects) and scale (books will include both fine-grained case studies and broad accounts of scientific cultures).
For readers, the series signals a new generation of scholarship captured in monograph form – tracking and analysing how science moves through our societies, cultures and lives. Employing innovative methodologies for investigating changing worlds is home to compelling new accounts of how science, technology, biomedicine and the environment translate and transform our social lives.

Previously published titles

Trust in the system: Research ethics committees and the regulation of biomedical research   Adam Hedgecoe

Personalised cancer medicine: Future crafting in the genomic era   Anne Kerr et al.

Embodiment and everyday cyborgs

Technologies that alter subjectivity

Gill Haddow

MANCHESTER UNIVERSITY PRESS

An electronic version of this book is also available
under a Creative Commons (CC-BY-NC-ND) licence,
thanks to the support of the Wellcome Trust, which
permits non-commercial use, distribution and reproduction
provided the author(s) and Manchester University Press
are fully cited and no modifications or adaptations are
made. Details of the licence can be viewed at
https://creativecommons.org/licenses/by-nc-nd/4.0

Published by Manchester University Press
Altrincham Street, Manchester M1 7JA

www.manchesteruniversitypress.co.uk

British Library Cataloguing-in-Publication Data
A catalogue record for this book is available from the British
Library

ISBN 978 1 5261 1418 1 hardback

First published 2021

The publisher has no responsibility for the persistence
or accuracy of URLs for any external or third-party
internet websites referred to in this book, and does not
guarantee that any content on such websites is, or will
remain, accurate or appropriate.

Typeset by Newgen Publishing UK

For David, Paige and Robyn.

Contents

Tables

Acknowledgements

There is a huge number of people that I owe equally huge debts of thanks to – in fact way too many to mention but I am going to try. My apologies to anyone that I have overlooked (in the faint hope that there is no one I have overlooked).

Back when I started writing I had two book buddies – Steve Kemp and Jane Calvert – whose input and thoughts were invaluable. Fast-forward and the most recent feedback was at the STIS Reading group where Morgan Currie, Miguel Garcia Sancho Sanchez, Michael Barany, Rob Smith, Rachel Simpson and Vassilis Galanos pushed me on to finish this book. I have been extremely fortunate to have the most amazing PhD students who all helped: Sara Bea, Fiona Coyle, Nathalie Dupin, Laura Donald, Leah Gilman, Vassilis Galanos, Anna Kuslits, Natalia Nïno, Janet Philp, Tirion Seymour, Anne Sorbie, Malissa Shaw, Rachel Simpson, Alison Wheatley and Laura Wigley and a final shout-out to José Goméz for reminding me about the Varela article!

The wonderful world of Science, Technology and Innovation Studies is an important home to be in and accepting of individuals like me who do not necessarily wear STS clothing all the time. Without the unstinting and unwavering support of Cathy Lyall, a person I am lucky to have as a friend, I would not have had the self-belief to persevere with writing. She is ever practical and always kind and I owe her too much. A corridor conversation with Cate Heeney reminded me that Descartes is still a thing! Niki Vermeulen's constant encouragement and generosity helped rehabilitate an interest in 3-D bioprinting and all things heart related.

Margaret Acton and Géraldine Debard were fantastic – each offering different input (the former of cake and the latter vocals on 'Electrifying Cyborg Heart'). It was Gé with whom I talked through how 'everyday cyborg' as a term might work. I am so grateful to Margaret for her proofreading skills, making this book a much easier experience for those reading it. The index in this book benefited from the magical skills of Moyra Forrest to whom I am eternally grateful.

During the writing of this book I was diagnosed with an autoimmune condition which made writing even more difficult than I had anticipated it would be. Then, of course, there is the impact that COVID-19 has had on everyone. Isabel Fletcher was a fantastic colleague and friend with a wicked sense of humour and was my fantastic wing commander when I was teaching. Without the support of my good friend and colleague, Fadhila Mazanderani, the journey would have been so much more difficult – I am truly fortunate to be able to work, study, argue, teach and sort out the plans for world domination with her. The research may never have seen the light of day until Tom Dark from Manchester University Press encouraged me to try and do this and then offered only patience and understanding when I missed several (all) deadlines.

From the wider intellectual field beyond STIS I benefited from reading and conversing with the likes of Alex Faulkner and John Gardner, Nelly Oudshoorn and cyborg scholar Chris Hables Gray. I had read his *Cyborg Handbook* years before the idea for this book was ever brought into being; I never imagined that I would be invited to contribute a short story based on my research with the everyday cyborgs to the follow-up book called '*Modified: Living as a Cyborg*' allowing me to experiment writing the fictional piece called '*When I first saw Jesus, he was a Cyborg*'. Muireann Quigley, through her enthusiastic support and belief in the concept of 'everyday cyborgs', helped me get to the final pages of this book and I am grateful to her that she is taking 'everyday cyborgs' onto a whole new register about the legal and ethical situations of cyborgisation. David Lawrence was a fun guy to be around and an intellectual ally. Klaus Hoëyer and his team in Copenhagen were incredibly generous, inviting me to explore with them mutual areas of interest and offering fantastic feedback which I benefited from enormously. I met Sam Taylor-Alexander, the first person to suggest the term 'everyday', however Sam passed away during the writing of this book and the world is not the same place without him. My fellow cyborg studies scholar, the wonderful Nelly Oudshoorn, was encouraging and shared her work and research with me. Donna McCormack offered wonderful insights into an earlier version of Chapter 1 when I was struggling with the gendering of organs.

I first started working with Shawn Harmon when we were both involved in the ESRC Innogen Centre in Edinburgh. Our partnership over the years since, whether it was art collaborations, writing journal articles or researching 'smart' technologies, was always stimulating and fun. This book wouldn't be where it is without benefiting from our collaborations. Among others with whom I worked alongside in the Mason Institute at the University of Edinburgh, Graeme Laurie was an inspiration and I learned a huge amount of what it means to be an academic in terms of kindness, openness and generosity. His ability to be constructive, never destructive, and his willingness to consider the best of everyone was a constant source of inspiration and I owe him more than he realises. The same also applies to Professor Sarah Cunningham-Burley who allowed me to take some risks as her Research Fellow and continued to support me. Thank you to the help given by Tirion Seymour the research fellow on this project.

If it hadn't been for Neil Grubb, the project that this book was based upon, namely 'Animal, Mechanical and Me: The Search for Replaceable Hearts', would have missed one of the most critical aspects of actually doing the research as he enabled the contact with implantable cardiac defribillator (ICD) patients and their families. It was Neil who alerted me to research that demonstrated ICDs were causing issues for some individuals and their families. Neil's team and others made me very welcome, and supported me always, despite the demanding nature of their positions in the UK National Health Service. My thanks also to the families who agreed to speak with me – to them I owe the largest debt of gratitude for their willingness to share their experiences, some of which were not always pleasant for them. They are the true stars of this book and it is their narratives and stories that have made this research what it is. I owe all of them thanks and by bringing their voices to the centre, I feel I have offered something by way of return. Maggie was inspirational and her willingness to document her feelings and allow them to be heard is what is great about the short film *Maggie's ICD*

Story. Without Maggie there would have been no 'Story' – her willingness to share her experiences was a massive act of generosity and courage and I will always be grateful to her.

None of this would have been possible if the Wellcome Trust had not offered funding for 'Animal, Mechanical and Me: The Search for Replaceable Hearts'. Not only did they fund the project for five years, but their University Award Scheme allowed me to secure an open contract at the University of Edinburgh. The stability that this position offered – in a period when so many individuals do not have that luxury – made me extremely fortunate. It offered an investment not only in the project itself but to the research that I am able to go forward with. Paul Woodgate, Dan O'Connor and Simon Chaplin offered unstinting encouragement.

One of the unique experiences I was able to have because of the Wellcome Trust funding was for a related engagement project: 'Everyday Cyborgs: Stories from the in/side Out'. It gave me an opportunity to take risks in terms of how art could offer a medium in which the social and ethical issues of human hybridity could be discussed. I was keen to ensure that individuals who are not usually consulted with about the social and ethical consequences of cyborgisation, xenotransplants and 3-D bioprinting had a role to play. Connecting with the people at North Edinburgh Arts such as the fantastic Kate Wimpress, Ali Grant and Allison Worth enabled the making of the film 'Broken Wings' with the young adults (Max, Siobhan, Mark, Liam, Annie and Mia). The time that the young people, and the artists who supported them, gave (Cameron, Claudine, Paddy and Sean) was incredible and took the project way beyond my expectations. It was one of my very best experiences and I hope they enjoyed it half as much as I did. My favourite fiction writer by far to work with is the wonderful Pippa Goldschmidt who has been a friend through thick or thin (through conceptual angst and expression overload). My second favourite (only kidding) is Ross Ziegelmeier. I am so grateful to him because without his creative talents *Maggie's ICD Story* as well as the animation *Everyday Cyborgs and Humanimals* would not have happened. My thanks to Cameron Duguid, an amazing artist and one of the nicest people I have met. My gratitude to Astrid Jaekel for allowing use of her wonderful images for the front cover of this book.

I would like to thank the reviewers of the many articles that I attempted to write and publish. I am glad that the Triad of I, the ambiguity of embodiment and biomedical nemesis made it through to the final cut. Any errors and mistakes are mine.

Like many who write books, I found the process, at first, more than a little tortuous and daunting, but it was a lot easier when surrounded by my family and friends. David, my partner in all things for over 25 years, helped me remain calm when I wanted drama, remaining my steady rock throughout all of this, and supporting me when I had limited energy and self-belief. My life is richer because of him. Finally, to my most amazing daughters – I can't put into words just quite how much you mean to me.

Gill Haddow, February 2021

Introduction: Animal, mechanical and me: Technologies that alter subjectivity

It is 1975, and I am 5 years old, waiting for my favourite TV pro-gramme to start. It is 'The Six Million Dollar Man' – an American TV series where the main character, Steve Austen (played by Lee Majors), undergoes surgery to repair and replace his limbs and organs with bionic prosthetics and cybernetic devices. The voice-over is saying these words: 'Gentlemen, we can rebuild him. We have the technology. We have the capability to make the world's first bionic man [sic]. Steve Austen will be that man. Better than he was before. Better. Stronger. Faster' (Voice-over to 'The Six Million Dollar Man', American TV Series, 1974–1978).

It is 2015, and I am interviewing Maggie, six weeks after she has had an implantable cardiac defibrillator (ICD) fitted in order to prevent her from having a sudden cardiac arrest (SCA). She shares with Steve Austen the fact that she too has to live a techno-organic hybrid life, allowing cybernetic systems to control some of her vital functions. Unlike Steve Austen, Maggie is not better, stronger or faster. This book is about individuals such as Maggie who are everyday cyborgs.

Introduction

In the UK, the present organ transplantation rate from deceased human donors does not meet the demand. This is a trend even in countries like Spain with comparatively high donation rates and an efficient procurement system. Improving transplantation rates by changes to the procurement system may be limited by the avail-ability of living or deceased human donors. Organ transplant-ation has been and always will be a victim of its own success. The more successful transplantation procedures have become, the more the actual number of organs that can be transplanted as well as a greater variety of organs that can be replaced. The shortage of deceased and living human donors is only likely to become more acute as the demand increases for a higher number and variety of human organs. Meeting the expansion of future needs for an ageing population suggests that attention must be given to alternative sources for organs as procurement systems such as opting-in or opting-out will not meet demand. To put it another way, more of us will require more in us.

Currently, highly experimental procedures such as xenotransplantation or 3-D bioprinting are touted as a means by which the persistent shortfall in human organs can be solved. For many years xenotransplantation has been heralded as having the potential to address the organ shortage. It involves taking organs from non-human animals and transplanting them into human recipients. At the moment pigs are generally preferred due to their organs being a comparable size to human organs, and allegedly raising fewer ethical concerns than using primates. However, despite using porcine valves to replace human heart structures, the replacement of entire human organs from non-human animals remains experimental and elusive. Xenotransplanted organs maintain their non-human animal cellular structure, which makes them liable to attack by the organ recipient's immune system. A more recent alternative is a proposal to 'regenerate organs'; these could be bioprinted from the cells of the recipient that requires them and this would make the donor the recipient and the recipient the donor. 3-D bioprinting works with organic materials (including living cells) from the individual to create structures approximating body parts (Vermeulen, Haddow, Seymour et al., 2017). Specialised printers use biological inks (bio-inks – such as differentiated stem cells, human embryonic stem cells or induced pluripotent stem cells to print layers of living materials one slice at a time, placing them on top of each other. It can avoid the challenges that xenotransplantation raises, for example, in terms of rejection and immunosuppression and associated ethical concerns with using non-human animals for transplantation.

Neither xenotransplantation nor 3-D bioprinting are successful alternative solutions for transplantation. Whereas xenotransplantation has been attempted in humans, it has proved largely unsuccessful and 3-D bioprinting of organs has yet to go to clinical trials.

I outline in more detail in Chapter 2 the challenges both have to overcome. I also offer some original research findings about how members of the public view a range of differing implantable bio-technologies to repair, replace or regenerate human body parts and the reasons for them.

Today human bodies are living in a society that is increasingly technologically mediated; people themselves are not just surrounded by information and communication technologies, but these are inserted within them (Hayles, 1995). '[W]hat is different in the 21st century about mechanical interventions is the scale on which devices are built and their coupling with electrical devices' as some highlight (Campbell, Clark, Loy et al., 2007: 231). Unlike the uptake of different *kinds* of organic materials that are living or deceased human or non-human animal, there are a range of different *types* of materials. Implantable medical technologies such as cochlear implants (CIs), deep brain stimulators (DBSs), in vivo biosensors (IVBs) and cardiac devices such as implantable cardiac devices (ICDs) and cardiac pacemakers (CPs) have features such as computational intelligence, autonomy and responsivity and can be defined as 'smart' (Haddow, Harmon and Gilman, 2016; Harmon, Haddow and Gilman, 2015). Viewed as the 'gold standard' in treatment of some heart conditions, ICDs are widely used in the UK and elsewhere. Most of the time, an ICD is dormant inside the body, only activating when it senses a heart arrhythmia (a fast heart beat). An ICD, will, for example, attempt to control heart beats and rhythms that are going too fast through a series of small electric shocks, called cardioversion. Failing cardioversion, an ICD will then produce a series of much stronger electric shocks, and it can go through this cycle several times until it has sensed a regular heart rate has been reinstated. The activity is stored as data and be communicated either in the clinic or from the individual's house, back to medical professionals based in the hospital. They are the 'informational stimulators communicating data about activity from the ICD within the person's body to hospital centres' (Bjorn and Markussen, 2013). Due to this ability, as well as being 'smart' insofar as it is an autonomous feedback function that detects a change in the body's cardiac environment, an ICD is a homeostatic closed feedback system. ICDs are a closed-loop feedback system and may be termed cybernetic, because of the control-command-communication-intelligence (C3I) features they incorporate (Haraway, 1991). Inserting cybernetic devices (cyb) into human organisms (org) creates a cyborg yet causes new types of biomedical vulnerabilities and has implications for subjectivity that will be the focus of Chapter 4. Should xenotransplantation and 3-D bioprinting then become successful, and dependent on apparent need, individuals may look forward to living their lives assisted internally with various montages of materials from origins as diverse as other humans, non-human animals or biomechanical (such as bionic, robotic or cybernetic). This future new normal of hybrid bodies is not necessarily an imagined one; it is a prediction that is partly based on current practices such as human transplantation and implantable medical technologies and possible developments such as xenotransplantation and 3-D bioprinting.

It could be argued that an ever increasing reliance on such biomedical solutions that are expensive and fast is creating a 21st-century identity crisis in modern Western societies. The identity crisis is due to the numerous and diverse creation of human hybrids. This hybridity is driven by the need for human beings to do everything in their power to avoid their demise. Over time, and as individuals age, their bodies will increasingly become a collage of organs and devices used to repair the structure and function of their viscera. Individuals will be less than 100 per cent human as they increasingly become augmented by different types and kinds of materials. The 'born body' of a human being, will become the exception rather than the rule and the 'techno-organic hybrid body' the new norm. Alterations to the body's integrity or, as I also refer to it, simply the 'insides' of the individual's body, causing it to become a hybrid, will have consequences for identity. Body modifications, even in our inside bodies, can result in alterations in subjectivity and the subsequent identity changes will partly be determined by the type and kind of material that is used to repair, replace or regenerate the body. In this book, I will outline the possible scale of the 21st-century identity crisis, by addressing the following:[1]

1   How do members of the public respond to hypothetical preferences for different *types* (mechanical) and *kinds* (non-human animal or human) of organs to repair the human body?

2   What are patient experiences of having undergone one type of body repair (such as implantable medical devices) and becoming an 'everyday cyborg'?
3   Consider why bodily modifications alter subjectivity, especially to the inside of the human body, and whether it is dependent on the origin of organs and devices.
4   Finally, bring social science research into dialogue with bio-medical and philosophical understandings of the connection between persons and their bodies, reflecting on this relationship as a fluid and dynamic experience whereby embodiment is always ambiguous.

I will be drawing on various philosophical and sociological theories about the relationship that is experienced between identity and the body.

For example, there is a well-known philosophical thought experiment called 'The Ship of Theseus' which considers how much of an object can be changed before it is no longer the same object. In this philosophical example, it is how much of a ship needs to be replaced before it is no longer the same ship. This philosophical question, applied to human beings, might be phrased as 'how much of a human being has to be replaced before that person is no longer the person they once were?' For example, Williams argues that in creating the cyborg it is 'best conceptualised on a continuum with the human organism at one end (i.e., the "all-human pole") and the pure machine (automaton) or artificial intelligence (AI) device at the other' (Featherstone and Burrows, cited in Williams, 1997: 1041). This depends on a view of the body as a quantitative sum of body parts, which is altered through the numerical addition of materiality. It is only the quantity that is important and not necessarily the quality. This leaves unexplored the question of what type of change might occur and with what artefacts. I want to answer this problem by tackling different but related questions such as 1) How does who we are relate to what we are? which therefore leads to 2) How does changing what we are affect who we are?

As well as reviewing empirical research that explores the narratives offered by organ transplant recipients, I will use findings from my research that I conducted with ICD patients, whom I will come to refer to as 'everyday cyborgs' (for reasons outlined further below). I also conducted focus group and survey research with various members of the UK public, the findings of which demonstrate clear preferences for real and hypothetical transplants and implants. In this research, I explore whether and how alterations to a human body from another human, from non-human animal or from mechanical origin alters subjectivity via a potential compromise of the insides and the integrity of the human body. By exploring how using different types and kinds of materials from different sources can have varied consequences for personal identity, the extent of the identity crisis can be evaluated as well as the strategies that individuals use to overcome them. The reliance on a technological 'fix' (in terms of addiction and solution) in relying on such sociotechnical means to solve health problems creates new vulnerabilities, for example, adjusting to new organic-technological hybridity as well as allowing cybernetics to be in control of body functions.

Who are we?

Philosophically, the connection a person has with their body can be traced back to the thinking of René Descartes in the seventeenth century and his idea that the body is a machine separate from the person. The body in Cartesian Dualism, is similar to the way that an individual might own or possess a car. Repairing the car has no effects on the driver. Modern-day practices such as organ donation and biomechanical implantation with smart and cybernetic devices are dependent on this view of the individual, their body and its organs. This view of a split between mechanical body and mind is based on the French philosopher's musings on the nature of knowledge. The result of his reflections was that the body is separated from the mind and the thinking self; Descartes' process of cognition produces his famous quote 'cogito, ergo sum' (I think, therefore I am). This Cartesian thinking is central to medical practice and also appears to have gained broader social acceptance. As Burkitt also argues, '[I]n the Western world individuals have grown accustomed to a way of understanding themselves which divides their existence between the mind and the body' (Burkitt, 1999: 7). Such a view of the inside of the human body is arguably cemented by the use of imaging technologies such as X-rays, cameras and scopes that can probe and visualise inside human flesh. Helman argues that the imagery produced by such medical interventions is associated mainly with the idea of the body as a mechanical entity:[2]

> The inside of the body is often conceived in the image of domestic plumbing coterminous with the view of the body as a machine. Many people think it is made up of a series of hollow cavities – called 'chest', 'stomach' or 'bladder' – connected with one another and with the orifices outside, by networks of piping or tubes. Diseases are seen as 'blockages' of one of these long soft tubes – an artery, a vein, a bronchus or a bowel. Such blocked tubes must be 'washed out' by laxatives, drugs or catheters, while the 'furred-up' arteries of the heart need to be regularly re-bored, or even 'by-passed,' by the mechanics of medical science.
>
> (Helman, 1991: 88)

The self as the brain?

In modern society, the mind or self is now closely associated with the brain as the materiality of self-identity and thinking as the process of cognition (Vidal, 2009). Indeed, recent attention focuses on interoception highlighting how the self is a neurological construct and sensation (Craig, 2002). This reinforces the Cartesian understanding of the relationship the self has with the body; the self is housed in the brain which is a distinct entity from the body, which itself is an alienable property from the rest of the body.

In Chapter 1, 'Ambiguous embodiment and organ transplantation', I show how this mechanistic Cartesian view of the self as being separate from the body is challenged by the existence of narratives about subjectivity alteration, that accompanied the beginnings of human organ heart transplantation. These stories suggest that for some organ transplant recipients, a change in their identity occurs after receiving the donated organ. In reviewing and comparing much of the early and later qualitative research with organ transplant recipients, a persistent theme of subjectivity alteration emerges, regardless of what organ is transplanted. Research by the anthropologists Fox and Swazey in the early days of heart transplantation, but also latterly in the work of Sharp (2006) and Shildrick (2015) with organ transplant recipients, demonstrates what is termed an 'anthropomorphisation' of the donated organ (Fox and Swazey, 1974, Fox and Swazey, 1992, Shildrick, 2014, Shildrick, 2015, Shildrick et al., 2009). Narratives emerging from interviews with organ donor recipients highlight common features such as a gender alteration or a feeling of youthfulness, but also inheriting behavioural and lifestyle preferences of the deceased donor, relating to music for example.

My intention is not to make claims about whether such stories are true or not; they are stories that are important to the individuals that share them and which have persisted from the beginnings of transplantation to the present day. Neither is it my desire to assess how many transplant recipients report them, as it is sufficient that such stories persist despite scepticism and alternative biomedical explanations. Rather I argue that these narratives from organ recipients are important because they bring into conversation the body and person, and a very different view of how a person experiences their body from the Cartesian Dualist one.

In his influential work *The Phenomenology of Perception*, written in 1945, Merleau-Ponty claims that we do not possess our bodies or are separate from them, as Descartes argues. We do not 'have' bodies, but we are our bodies (Merleau-Ponty, 2012). For Merleau-Ponty, a body is the sensory gate into and onto the physical world. It is both object and subject in a relationship of perception with the environment. All our experience of the world is therefore embodied. In the arguments of Merleau-Ponty, modifications to the body, either as a loss or addition, can alter subjectivity.[3] Merleau-Ponty uses the example of an object such as a man's cane or a woman's feather in her hat, both 'expresses the power we have of dilating our being in the world, or of altering our existence through incorporating new instruments' (Merleau-Ponty, 2012: 145). Post-phenomenological perspectives, especially the work of Ihde, discuss our embodied relations with technology and the way that technology mediates the perception of the world (Ihde, 1990). Similarly, in his book *Natural Born Cyborgs*, author Andy Clark suggests that most humans were born to be cyborgs, not because of any traditional 'physical wire-and-implant mergers, so much as on our openness to information-processing mergers' (Clark, 2003: 6). Clark views tools, such as pens, papers, watches and so on as being 'mind-enhancing technologies' (Clark, 2003: 7). However, as Clark stresses, these technologies are not actual changes to the human body in the same way as an amputation or implanted devices are and therefore may not speak directly to the consequences for identity or subjectivity when integrity is breached and the inside of the body modified. The phenomenological 'embodiment as the (perceptual) experience' is important but I am arguing for something slightly different and that is how the *experience of embodiment* is altered by amputation, transplantation and implantation of technoscience.

Thus the relationship a person has with their body, generally referred to as the experience of embodiment, is ambiguous as a person both is a body (in terms of phenomenological understanding of 'I am a body') and has a body (in terms of a Cartesian Dualist understanding of 'I have a body). The research and thinking offered in this book highlight that having or being a body, of embodiment, is not a static state, however, but a fluid experience. I suggest that the ambiguity is not just in terms of *whether* I am, or I have a body, but its fluidity is based on events that bring about questions of *when* I am, or I have a body. That moment occurs when events such as implantation and transplantation are acted upon the body, bringing the ambiguity of embodiment, to the forefront of the experience. This is not a new idea. The construction of identity is a process, for example, that is disrupted by illness (Charmaz, 1995) and also as Sulik discusses, by technoscience innovations (Sulik, 2011). What I am adding to these discussions is a consideration of how modifications to the integrity of the body also has consequences for identity.

Is it self and a person then?

Contrary to an on-going emphasis on neurological identity that promotes a discourse of the self, located in the brain, there is more to embodiment than an individual as a brain and as an owner of a body. It is undeniable that the self is crucial for experiencing personal reflection. Indeed, it is current in everyday language to be able to 'look inside yourself', 'search for your inner self', 'find yourself' and so on. The practice of mindfulness involves taking time to gather and pay attention to the thoughts that are experienced as being located in the head. Certainly, the idea of mindfulness has recently gained attention with an emphasis on the practice of awareness and of 'being' in the moment (Williams and Penman, 2014). Mindfulness is a form of meditation on the senses of sight, touch, hearing, smell and taste. It is a way of becoming reconnected and of 'waking up to what's happening inside of you, and in the world, moment by moment' (Williams and Penman, 2014: 39). Most of the discussion in this book draws on authors that include and refer to the idea of self.

I prefer to use words such as identity, person or subjectivity as a way to indicate that I am not focusing on the self, insofar as this is understood as purely cognitively based or perceptually focused in terms of a phenomenological ideology. I wish to avoid using the word self, in favour of using subjectivity or identity as both allude to the more diffuse elements of the personal which is often experientially bodily based and as I then develop can also be relational due to interactions with other people. By identity and subjectivity, I mean the way that an individual experiences herself as embodied. Subjectivity indicates a going beyond the conceptualisation of embodiment as Cartesian Dualism and as a self only having a body. Moreover, identity is different to the phenomenologically based embodiment as perception, because identity focuses on the experience of embodiment (and not embodiment as experience). Additionally, using identity as important in the experience of embodiment recognises that a person's body has an inside as well as its outside body.

Dead or alive? Mine, yours or something else altogether?

Given the emphasis I have placed on considering the experience of embodiment as being ambiguous, and that this experience includes alterations to the inside of the body and its integrity, I turn in Chapter 2 to how body modifications occurring inside the body can alter subjectivity. I hope to do this by answering the question of whether implantation of different materials, whether in kind (animal or human) or type (mechanical), are said or thought to cause different types of subjectivity alteration My research included four focus groups, followed by a survey questionnaire with young people. I asked people about their hypothetical preferences for different *kinds* of materials originating from different origins (such as from living or deceased human organ donation, non-human animal sources such as xenotransplantation or even from the same body as in 3-D bioprinting) as well as different *types* of materials such as implantable devices.

In the questionnaire, the young people were offered these different kinds and types of materials as options to be ranked in terms of what they would hypothetically most like and what would be the least liked. The results of this research demonstrate that participants in both the focus groups and the questionnaire found xenotransplantation the most unpopular by far. Dislike for xenotransplantation was related to the ethics of treatment and use of non-human animals, physiological, functional and immunological compatibility, as well as implications for the individual as a person, and human beings as a species. When pig's organs are placed inside a human body, it creates a hybrid entity that transgresses the familiar and taken-for-granted boundaries about what is human and what is not, blurring the boundary between species (Chakrabarty, 2003, Alter, 2007, Robert and Baylis, 2003). Although pig's organs are comparable in size to human ones, pigs provoke negative reactions in the focus groups and survey responses, because of the pig's association with dirt. A pig's organ, it was imagined, could make the person more 'pig-like'. Pigs are thought to be unclean, and their usage in transplants challenges known schemata of what it is to be a 'pig' and what it is to be 'human', in a way that organs from another individual or other human beings do not. Xenotransplants are thought to flout the socially constructed natural boundaries between species and provokes a 'yuck' reaction. This can be linked to ideas about pollution, captured by Mary Douglas, as behaviour that 'is the reaction which condemns any object or idea likely to confuse or contradict cherished classifications' as out-of-place (Douglas, 1966: 36). I will also relate pollution behaviour to Kass' (2002) 'wisdom of repugnance'.

This socio-cultural rejection may be as challenging to overcome as the human biological rejection of any foreign organ.

On the other hand, the popularity of 3-D bioprinting as the most preferred option highlights the importance of the similarity of materiality: that is, of having the perceived quality of sameness and compatibility in terms of the human. That is, the origin from a familiar subjectivity (the importance of the person themselves or others close to them), and species compatibility (of other humans). Hence, the next popular choices were a known living human donor, followed by an organ from a deceased stranger. All these human replacements were the most popular, and reflects somewhat the importance of the familiar human and of close personal links or biological ties. Living donors are generally known to the recipient; therefore, it is possible to know the precise origin of the organ. Not just that it is an organ from another human but that it is an organ from a known and familiar human. These findings suggest, therefore, a clear preference for human organ replacements to be sourced from the same person; next, a familiar person; followed by a similar individual (e.g. other human bodies).

In Chapter 2, hypothetical views about implantable devices dem-onstrate lower popularity than human organ transplantation but are not as unpopular as xenotransplantation. Fears around infec-tion and malfunctioning technology were given as concerns and those who said they least preferred mechanical implants articulated concerns about the repercussions for subjectivity, with ideas of becoming robotic or fears of being more machine-like being given. Those who were in favour of mechanical implants emphasised how the modification would alter their identity, turning them into the cyborgs such as those portrayed in literature and film, for example 'Robocop', and androids portrayed in science-fiction films such as 'Terminator'. The ambiguity of embodiment emerges in various ways and degrees of subjectivity alteration when exploring preferences for different technological and organic materials to be embodied. In sum, I shall argue that although individuals are embodied, they are also embedded, in various social contexts that construct meanings associated with what is human/non-human animal, male/female, or organic/non-organic and although this is obviously projected onto the visible surface of the body the process also occurs in the inside body. Gender appears as a highly porous narrative, as do features thought to characterise non-human animals such as what a pig is. At the end of Chapter 2, I discuss how the concept of *contamination* or *contagion* as socio-cultural terms can be used to explain why it is that particular social characteristics are attached to the narratives of a human or non-human organ. Contamination is based on the mechanism of transferring characteristics as told by those who have experienced human organ transplantation, and imagined by those who consider how they might experience non-human implantation or transplantation.

Who is afraid of the cyborg? All of us

The data presented in Chapter 2 demonstrate strong preferences about not modifying the integrity of the human body with non-human materials and concerns are articulated about breaching individual subjectivity as well as transgressing the species boundaries. Hypothetical views about implantable devices demonstrate lower popularity than human organ transplantation but are not as unpopular as xenotransplantation. Fears around infection and malfunctioning technology were given as concerns and those who said they least preferred mechanical implants articulated concerns about the repercussions for subjectivity; with ideas of becoming robotic or fears of being more machine-like being given. Those who were in favour of mechanical implants emphasised how the modification would alter their identity turning them into the cyborgs such as those portrayed in literature and film, e.g. 'Robocop' and androids portrayed in science-fiction films such as 'Terminator'. Yet just how relevant are these views to individuals who live with implanted devices?

In Chapter 3, 'Reclaiming the cyborg', I continue to suggest there is a need for an embodied approach to technology as well as a closer analysis of what this intimate techno-organic hybrid body means to subjectivity. That is, given embodiment is ambiguous, what are the consequences for subjectivity when a person's relationship to their body is altered via an active, smart implantable medical device?

From Chapter 3 onwards, the ICD and its role in creating everyday cyborgs is the focus of the rest of the book. Whereas the first half of the book focuses upon human organ transplantation and preferences for other transplantations and implantations, the second half draws attention to the experiences of living with a device implanted into the body.

However, using the term 'cyborg' as a way to describe people is controversial due in large part to the cyborg's depiction in the genres of science and horror fiction. This is because as Turkle notes: '[W]e approach our technologies through a battery of advertising and media narratives; it is hard to think above the din' (Turkle, 2011). In the public imagination the cyborg is a science-fiction monster born in the image of a technologically enhanced organism as portrayed in a multitude of books and films (Oetler, 1995). Often the distinction between cyborgs, androids and robots is conflated. Robots are fully mechanical artificial sophisticated devices with no organic elements, whereas an android is a robot that bears an external resemblance to a human or non-human living organism. A cyborg is a contraction of the words cybernetic and organism. Placing a cybernetic technology into an organism, as shown in a science-fiction or horror genre, nega-tively affects the individual's subjectivity. These cyborg monsters are visible techno-organic hybrids typically but not always, shown as being incapable of *feeling* or demonstrating emotions. Somehow the addition of a cybnernetic technology creates a less human body and a subjectivity that is inhumane. A feature that was imagined as bene-ficial by some of the young adult survey respondents.

The 'cybernetic' label I use, however, fits within the original definition of the cyborg, which was used in the 1960s to describe the bodily modifications required to create a homeostatic feed-back system for 'men' to survive future space exploration in hos-tile environments (Clynes and Kline, 1960). In its original use, the cyborg was a means to describe the physiological adaptations that future space travel would need (Clynes and Kline, 1960).

Implanting devices avoids the subjectivity alterations that organic parts may cause the recipient. Mechanical parts have no associ-ation with the once living and are not contaminated by them, and cannot in turn, therefore, contaminate the recipient. Whereas organ transplants can cause episodes of rejection, implantable devices are associated with malfunction and infection. In Chapter 3 and Chapter 4, I take a closer look at the issues inserting cybernetics into the body cause their recipients and show how these do not make them inhuman as more commonly associated with science-fiction monsters. On the contrary, it makes them more vulnerable and more human. The lives of grinders and biohackers, and others who prefer to modify through do-it-yourself implants, are not dependent upon or controlled by their implants and are not made vulnerable by their body modifications (Warwick, 2003, Warwick, 2004). Riding a bike or swallowing a pill does not create a cyborg either. Even though those that originally coined the term 'cyborg' might argue that such activities can make you a 'simple cyborg' (Clynes and Kline, 1960), it would not fit in the narrow definition offered in this book that takes a much tighter definition of a cyborg. It is narrowly defined through stressing the cybernetic system involved, however it is simultaneously expansive enough to allow other forms of implantable medical technologies. Implanted medical devices are relied upon by medical professionals and patients alike, offering the possibilities of increases in the length and quality of lives. While a broad understanding of the term 'implantable' might include those technologies that are consumed (e.g. pharmaceuticals), such products are not intended to be permanently incorporated as an active medical device is which is placed inside the body. I would also exclude other implantable medical technologies such as prosthetics or hip joints that do not, arguably, have the features of a cybernetic device and I use Haraway's (1991) 3CI – command, control and communication-intelligence. For example, an active medical device is an instrument, which, with its software, can be used for diagnostic and therapeutic purposes, relying on a power source other than that generated by the body.

Other versions of cybernetic

Colleagues and I have suggested that implantable medical technologies can have different levels or forms of current 'smart' or 'cybernetic' technologies (Haddow, Harmon and Gilman, 2016). In our previous research, we suggested that 'smart' technologies can carry a 'sting', or rather multiple stings relating to, on the one hand, being complex, autonomous and responsive, and on the other side, igniting concerns about lack of control and vulnerability (Haddow, Harmon and Gilman, 2016; Harmon, Haddow and Gilman, 2015). The ICD in particular has the potential to alter the recipient's subjectivity and identity through creating a hybrid techno-organic body that is being controlled by a cybernetic system. Cybernetic technology does not cause a chronic case of dehumanisation as envisioned in popular culture and literature despite modifications to the human body, making it less human in organic terms.

On the contrary, a *cyborgisation is about the reconfiguration of humanisation caused by the vulnerability*. However, the term 'cyborg' has cultural and literary infamy that does not allow space for its use to describe individuals. This fallacy of 'dehumanisation' through cyborgisation is inherited from the creation of the cyborg as a male science-fiction monster. Creating and existing as an everyday cyborg cannot be any more different from the portrayal of celluloid on the emotionless and inhumane cyborg monster. Instead, the everyday cyborg becomes more vulnerable, despite becoming less human in a new techno-organic hybrid form.

Since Haraway published her 'Cyborg Manifesto', the use of medical technologies that augment and replace human organs and limbs has increased exponentially, and improved dramatically, resulting in increasing numbers of people becoming, to all and intents and purposes, cybernetic organisms. For Haraway, the cyborg is a 'cybernetic organism, a hybrid of machine and organism, a creature of social reality as well as a creature of fiction' (1991: 119). Haraway's cyborg has an ability to liberate individuals from classification. The cyborg is a challenge to us to break away and accept that we have responsibility for the cages we have constructed of who and what we are. Haraway argues this is not about focusing purely on the technology per se, but upon the socially structured relations amongst people that have been historically constituted (1991: 165). As Haraway suggests although 'we may be all cyborgs', I suggest that it is time to draw attention to who exactly the 'we' are.

Few studies examine how the 'cyborg' condition is created as an empirical entity, and as such, this book offers unique insights into life with a heart device. Scholars have suggested terms such as 'ICD cyborg' (Oudshoorn, 2015, Oudshoorn, 2016) or the 'mundane cyborg' (Mentor, 2011), and this body of research is making significant contributions to the emerging field of cyborgisation. For instance, in Chapter 3, I expand Oudshoorn's term the 'ICD cyborg' as she uses it to refer to the participants in her research. For reasons that I detail further in Chapter 3, I introduce the term 'everyday' to highlight cybernetic technologies such as ICDs, which as technoscientific innovations are increasingly relied upon daily by clinicians and health professionals to save lives. The 'everyday' encompasses the increase in medically created cyborgs while highlighting the day-to-day activity of routine. And is also about the extraordinary experiences of living as a cyborg when life itself cannot be taken for granted (Das, 2010).

As I will argue in more detail in Chapter 3, the inclusion of the prefix 'everyday' is essential as it offers analytical purchase in studying variation in those who experience differing cyborgisation processes. The usefulness of the 'everyday cyborg' would consider the conditions the cybernetic system was inserted in, where and what for, the permanence of the device and the possibility of removal, as well as the complexity of its functionality and ultimately who benefits. The term 'everyday cyborg' is made vulnerable from cyborgisation, and the term 'everyday' answers the plea to examine less attractive technoscience options made by Timmermans and Berg that: 'in the seemingly "technical" matters that deeply relevant, social issues are "hidden" – such as inclusion/exclusions of certain groups or voices, of the subtle restructuring of patients' or professionals' identities' (2003: 108). By reclaiming the cyborg for the daily routine, social issues that are previously 'hidden' can be made visible.[4]

So, one of the 'hidden' aspects is the way current surgical practices reflect technological developments that do not challenge existing inequalities in cyborg society but reify and amplify them. Hence, the value of the term the 'everyday cyborg' encompasses the process of social stratification in cyborgisation that benefits one sub-section of the population over another. That is, as I shall show later in the book, the everyday cyborg that is created through the insertion of a cybernetic technology such as ICDs are generally male. The term 'everyday cyborg' is needed therefore to highlight how the practice of cyborgisation in hospital operating theatres are creating fewer female everyday cyborgs than males, reflecting male cyborg dominance in literature and culture, as well as in day-to-day life. The everyday cyborgs are created within social structures that reflect developments and practices and are therefore reifying but not (yet) challenging, existing inequalities in a cyborg society.

Cyborg vulnerability

In a future in which (some) individuals may become cyborg, more attention needs to be paid to the lived experience of living with technology that has increasing autonomy over and in our bodies. Reclaiming the 'cyborg' term allows a more thoroughgoing and wide-ranging discussion about the vulnerabilities created by implanting cybernetic devices into human bodies (Oudshoorn, 2016). ICDs can cause their (albeit male) cyborgs and their significant others emotional, physiological, psychological and social challenges that are rarely made visible. A cyborg identification thus reawakens interest in a techno-organic hybrid condition, leading to understandings about the new obstacles and vulnerabilities that are created. And as Oudshoorn argues, these new forms of vulnerabilities emanate from within the human body (Oudshoorn, 2016).

Using the voices of the everyday cyborgs in Chapter 4, 'Everyday cyborgs and the love-hate cybernetic relationship', I describe the day-to-day experiences that living as a cyborg involves and what this reconfiguration of vulnerable humanisation entails. Everyday cyborgs and their significant others have important stories to share about the varying initial reactions, and subsequent acclimatisation to, living with ICDs. In 2014, throughout a two-year period, I conducted 21 face-to-face interviews with everyday ICD cyborgs in Scotland, UK.[5] With National Health Service (NHS) ethical approvals, participants were recruited using NHS gatekeepers and a consent-to-consent approach. Using interview data from 21 everyday cyborgs and 13 of their significant others, I argue that everyday cyborgs face unique challenges that separate them from other cardiac patients. Despite the vast amount of research reported on enhanced life function and improved quality of life, some research suggests 'living the hybrid life' via cardiac devices has detrimental effects on some recipients (Green and Moss, 1969, Tchou et al., 1989, Luderitz, et al., 1994, Sakensa, 1994, Duru et al., 2001, Burns et al., 2005, Kuhl et al., 2006, Birnie et al., 2007, Pedersen et al., 2008, Magyar-Russell et al., 2011, Marshall, Ketchell and Maclean, 2011, Yuhas et al., 2012, Vriesendorp et al., 2013). In all cases, this is an existence whereby the everyday cyborgs and their families need support through the adaptations required for the cybernetic changes in embodiment and social life.

I go into detail about the love/hate relationship the everyday cyborgs told me that they have for their ICD. These challenges to living a techno-organic hybrid life can be summarised as: 1) acclimatising to an alien(ating) device that involves it becoming a 'part of the body' and 2) reconciling to being under the control of the ICD.

On becoming a cyborg: living the techno-organic hybrid life

For the everyday cyborgs, it is the paradox of intimacy that is created as the cybernetic device within the body also creates distance (as they cannot reach it) and a lack of control (as its functioning cannot be altered by the everyday cyborg either). In creating the techno-organic hybrid form of a cyborg, the body modification involved is a technological addition. The narratives about techno-logical devices do not evoke the porosity or contamination as those about organic materials. The stories focus more on how the everyday cyborg 'humanises' or makes the ICD a 'part of them'. As stories from the everyday cyborgs (outlined in Chapter 4) show, the ICD's alien presence is caused by breaching the integrity of the body during its implantation. From then, the ICD continues to be present on both the inside (it is inside-out) and outside (from the outside-in). The sensation of the ICD being on the inside, as well as a skin silhouette on the outside, reminds the everyday cyborg an 'alien' has breached the integrity and image of their body existing inside their bodies. Cyborgisation therefore makes the body's absence that is a feature of everyday living become absent or in Leder's terms a 'dys-appearance' (1990). An acclimatisation to the cyborgisation process is to a new techno-organic hybrid identity, and strategies are required to overcome vulnerability to cybernetic technology. The area of the chest where the ICD exists becomes a focal point for the everyday cyborg. For the everyday cyborg, the absent absences of the body and organs are not static states but variable, e.g. when the body heals the ICD becomes slowly enmeshed into the body creating a more comfortable form of techno-organic hybridity. Everyday cyborgs live with a machine inside their bodies that they can feel from the inside out; there was a strong sensation of the ICD being inside the body. For most, most of the time, the sensation was not dwelt upon and the body is, as Leder (1990) would suggest, an absence in the same way as the rest of the viscera are. Acclimatisation to hybridity occurs when the ICD's body presence becomes an absent absence, and the body returns to an absent state. This involves the cybernetic device becoming made into a 'part of the person' – a body addition that becomes part of their identity, integrity and image. Ironically, despite the everyday cyborgs' inability to reach their device, the communication feature of the ICD might leave the everyday cyborg vulnerable to hacking into the device. In other words, cyborgisation can make the body vulnerable and is a vulnerability emitting from both the inside-out and the outside-in. This ability to interfere with the device's ability to function or in accessing the data is currently dwelt upon by regulatory organisations and policymakers. Little is known about how individuals who are implanted with such features perceive such threats (Haddow, Harmon and Gilman, 2015). I outline the everyday cyborgs' views on the possibility of hacking and show these concerns were reported as not relevant to them.

Vulnerability from the cybernetic device within

As per the issue of unauthorised access and adjusting to a new techno-organic hybridity, the second way a new vulnerability results from cyborgisation is rooted in the specific capacity of the ICD to deliver a powerful electric shock, physically compromising the everyday cyborg. This is a shock in both meanings of the word 'shock', referring to its suddenness and that it comes from an electrical source. Indeed, studies have repeatedly shown that anxiety is heightened in patients whose ICDs have fired compared to those who have not experienced shocks (Hegel et al., 1997, Dougherty, 1995). The electric shock treatment that the ICD emits is noted to be the most distressing aspect of treatment for many. The shock that the ICD emits is shocking both in terms of the pain that it causes as well as the unexpectedness of its occurrence. Oudshoorn suggests that '[H]aving a machine inside your body without knowing when or where it may jolt you induces feelings of disbelief and anxiety', leading her to discuss the new vulnerabilities that ICDs cause

(2016: 8). In her analysis of ICD patient internet support pages, Oudshoorn (2015) notes the ICD is a device that acts outwith the control of the patient, and is an implantation that is rarely reversed. Oudshoorn also interviewed 14 individuals with ICDs (as well as conducting observations at the clinics during check-ups), suggesting that cyborgisation leads to new types of vulnerability 'as an internal rather than an external threat and as harm you may try to anticipate but can never escape' (Oudshoorn, 2016: 267). The findings from my research complement this body of work and suggest that there are strategies to overcome the vulnerability created by a new techno-organic hybrid identity which the everyday cyborg uses to allow acclimatisation:

1   How the techno-organic hybrid embodiment is acclimatised to depends on whether the ICD is perceived to be a supportive aid. This reconciliation needs a change from seeing the ICD as doing harm to the everyday cyborg, to switching to experiencing it as doing something for them. In a similar way that the ICD become part of their body, the ICD is a benefit in their lives.
2   Most of the everyday cyborgs who were shocked explained how it was *their* actions causing the ICD to fire (whether it was by excess exercise, consumption or concern) thus re-inserting their control over the ICD firing.

Eventually, and for some periods, the ICD is no longer a source of alienation, and it becomes accepted as a part of the everyday cyborg's body image and integrity, of their identity and of their lives (that includes others around them).[6] Being an everyday cyborg, then, is a fluid experience of 'dys-appearance' – of being aware and focused on embodiment as a techno-organic hybrid after implantation and post-activation, and then of this status becoming an absence – as the everyday cyborg acclimatises and the ambiguity of embodiment is no longer relevant. The issues around the body disappear to be replaced with normal living (Sobchack, 2010, Leder, 1990).

The biomedical nemesis

The intimacy between technology and organism has a particular rehumanising effect from living the techno-organic hybrid life and seeking control over a cybernetic technology that can be seen and felt but cannot be reached or removed. Concluding in Chapter 5, I refocus on the accounts of altered subjectivity and compare the materials from non-human animal, mechanical and human. That is, how respondents expect to take on characteristics of their human or non-human animal donor; and then how recipients relate their experiences of cybernetic technologies that require strategies of acclimatisation (overcoming body hybridity and vulnerability caused by the device). For example, the ICD is an alien effect and a body modification that changes the body and alters subjectivity in a less porous way than a human organ transplant does, or a xeno-transplant is predicted to do. With technological additions such as the ICD, the risk to subjectivity is not that of becoming more like the donor (e.g. human or non-human animal). Quite obviously, there is no donor to become like. It is not the case that because of the technological artefact and a creation of techno-organic hybrid body, making the individual's body less human, that this causes an alteration in subjectivity to one that makes them less emotional, caring and humane, as is depicted in the process of cyborgisation in literary or cultural narratives. In contrast to the popular depiction of cyborgisation as being dehumanising, the everyday experience of cyborgisation is of vulnerability and rehumanisation.

The increasing reliance on technoscientific processes may be a case of a much wider process of 'biomedicalisation'; a state that is different to, but is sprung from medicalisation for the modern age. Biomedicalisation refers to 'the increasingly complex, multisited, multidirectional processes of medicalization that today are being reconstituted through the emergent social forms and practices of a highly and increasingly technoscientific biomedicine' (Clarke et al., 2010: 162). I argue that due to a reliance on the technoscientific 'fix' (in terms of addiction and solution), it is creating an identity crisis that is part of living in an increasing 'hypercapitalist, techno-manic' society (Valente, 2011). Inspired by Illich's (Illich, 2003) medical nemesis, whereby medicalisation is the treatment for the diseases that medicalisation itself creates, so it is with technological and cybernetic fixes creating a biomedical nemesis. In as much as there was never any actual choice to be made between animal, mechanical and human, for some, there was never an element of choice in becoming a cyborg.

Notes

1 From 2013–18, I conducted a sociological study in the UK, funded by the Wellcome Trust, called 'Animal, Mechanical and Me: The Search for Replaceable Hearts' of which I say more later.
2 It is interesting to note that the term visceral can mean having deep feelings about something that is not necessarily based on reason (as well as pertaining to the fleshy insides of the human body).
3 Shildrick argues that a phenomenological approach to organ transplantation introduces a harm being done both to the unity and identity of individuals:

> Once a phenomenological approach to any organ donation – Western or non-Western alike – is undertaken, then all sorts of difficult questions begin to emerge that should at least make us reconsider the assumed benefit of transplantation procedures. The problematic of the assault on a body's putative unity and self-identity – whatever form that takes in the social imaginary – cannot be set aside in favour of positivistic representations of biomedical advance.
>
> (Shildrick, M. 2010. Some Reflections on the Socio-cultural and the Bioscientific Limits of Bodily Integrity. *Body & Society*, 16, 11–22)

4 Others who have adopted the term 'everyday cyborg' use it more broadly, but as equally important so to interrogate legal issues such as ownership and risk (Quigley and Ayihongbe, 2018).
5 One participant preferred to share his experiences through e-mail and this information is not reported.
6 Indeed, I discuss Dalibert's research findings, which suggest there is an acclimatisation or incorporation process necessary to adjust to a deep brain stimulator. This is based on the individual's acceptance of the technology as being 'part of them', but can also be affected by intercorporeal relationships with others (Dalibert, 2016).

1

Ambiguous embodiment and organ transplantation

> Recipients of cadaver organs, like those with organs from living relatives, often express the sentiment that one can acquire the donor's emotional, moral, or physical characteristics. Such qualities can be elaborate and imaginative, especially when the donor was an anonymous stranger. Some patients live in fear of the independent or animate qualities of the new organs.
>
> (Sharp, 1995: 372)

Introduction

This first chapter aims to offer an introduction to the stories told by organ transplant recipients that relate to how they experienced a subjectivity[1] alteration post-transplant. Clinical organ transplantation between human beings has been done for the last 50 years and is no longer the experimental treatment that it once was. Organ transplantation depends on a view of human bodies being machine-like and forming a separate container for the self, perhaps akin to an individual driving a car. Although this body-as-machine view is relied upon by medical professionals and is one that medical procedures such as organ transplantation are dependent upon, the persistence of alternative stories of bodies and organs suggest a more complex relationship exists between a person and the body.

As I shall outline below, narratives of subjectivity alteration can be found in interviews as far back to the first heart transplant Louis Washkansky underwent in the late 1960s. Such narratives persist decades later, for example, in a book written by Claire Sylvia (1997) called *A Change of Heart: The Extraordinary Story of a Man's Heart in a Woman's Body*. She details the subjectivity alterations she experienced after receiving an organ from a young boy called Tim: changes that were experienced by her before knowing anything about the donor and yet which coincided with the donor characteristics.

It is difficult to ascertain how many organ transplant recipients report some form of subjectivity change and certainly not every transplant recipient does. Nevertheless, even if it is not a widespread phenomenon, it is an entrenched one. It is not my intention to challenge whether these stories are true or not. On the contrary, I think these narratives are important and I wish to explore what subjectivity alteration tells us about how individuals experience embodiment. That is, whether an individual has a body which they are separate from as the body-as-machine model suggests, or whether a person experiences embodiment as being a body and there is no separation. Or indeed whether the experience of embodiment is ambiguous, variable and fluid, affected by events occurring in the body, and the environment outside it.

Through a review of social science research conducted with organ transplantation recipients, it is shown that the identity changes most frequently mentioned are an alteration in gender or age, or preferences for food or music. Medical and social science communities have long sought to offer explanations for these stories, and these relate to social theories about contagion and contamination and biological explanations about the existence of cellular memory. These explanations differ in explaining how the characteristics are transferred (whether it is biological and cellular or social contamination). I suggest that because donated organs come from another human being, there is a shared understanding of what it is to be a human being that is universal, but being a human can be a particular version of this universality. There are a variety of ways of being human, so this generates many different characteristics about the person who donated the organs and the origin of human organs; for example, they came from an individual who was a certain age or gender, to a preference for particular foods. Narratives such as these relating to the universality but the individuality of the human organs suggest the organ is not a culturally or socially neutral entity in the same way as an implantable device might be (as I go on to discuss later in Chapter 4).

In this chapter, I outline the narratives of organ transplant recipients, that tell of how receiving an organ changes who they are and alters their subjectivity. The donated organ is, in some way, rehumanised or socialised with the donor's presence (Fox and Swazey, 1992). This challenges a Cartesian Dualism ideology that suggests the body and the person are separate and distinct entities. Turning towards a more phenomenological approach originating from Merleau-Ponty (2012, 1945), and later by Leder (1990), I compare accounts of subjectivity alteration in transplantation and amputation to delve further into what happens to identity when modifications are made to the body a person was first born with. Organ transplant recipients can gain a new identity whereas amputating limbs is synonymous with an identity loss – the first procedure occurs inside the human body and is an invisible gain, whereas the latter is a visible loss. I introduce the concept of the 'Triad of I' to highlight just how important the integrity of the human body is, both to identity and body image. I show how assumptions are made about the biological characteristics of the donated organs based on the donor's gender identity. The donated organ is considered to be coterminous with the gender of the donor, despite the organs not being visible.

I begin, however, with the history of organ transplantation as a procedure, and then I turn to a thoroughgoing review of what 'organs with history' can say about how the body and its organs are experienced.

Inner space and outer face

Of any transplant that would entail an alteration of a person's subjectivity or identity, a face transplant would appear to the most challenging for the recipient. The recipient's face will become a hybrid of both their face and that of the donor and not a true reflection of either. For the recipient, however, the donated face is a constant and visible reminder that the facial modification is a visible alteration in identity. Isabelle Dinoire received the first face transplant in 2005.[2] She reported that the face transplant had been challenging to cope with due to several cases of rejection caused by the ability of a human body's immune system to attack that which is perceived as foreign. As she also outlines in her book *Le Baiser d'Isabelle*, there was also the strange sensation of accepting the inside of 'someone else's mouth. It was odd to touch, to touch it with my tongue. It was soft. It was horrible' (quoted in *The Guardian* 2007).[3] There are many arguments around the ethics, cost, and long-term health implications of a non-life-saving procedure such as facial transplantation, the perceived vulnerability of the patients, a lack of donor anonymity, patient compliance and the effect on the recipient's social circle and so on. A key concern relates to the way that the face reflects personal identity:

> As an expressive part of our body, it represents identity in a way no other part of the body does. It is the most intimate, the most individual characteristic of our body. It is what we recognise as ourselves and what others recognise as us.
>
> (Freeman and Abou Jaoude, 2007: 76)

The question that drove much of the debate in the first face transplant appeared to be about whether or not transplantation had gone too far in altering the identity of the person (Taylor-Alexander, 2004, Freeman and Abou Jaoude, 2007, Le Breton, 2015, Theodorakopoulou et al., 2017, Martindale and Fisher, 2019). However, similar concerns about identity were raised when the first heart transplant was conducted almost 40 years previously. If the face is the image of identity, then the heart is the internal site of identity, as it is an organ culturally most closely associated with the intangible aspects of what emotions, soul and personhood are. Therefore, as I turn to next, transplanting the heart might also be thought to have profound consequences for a person's identity.

The first heart transplant

It is 3 December 1967. The South African heart surgeon, Christiaan Barnard (1922–2001) has just conducted the world's first heart transplant. He did so by removing the heart from 25-year-old Denise

Darvall who had died in a car accident and placing it into the body of grocer Louis Washkansky. Louis, perhaps like others before him who are the 'first' in experimental procedures, died only 18 days later. His death from pneumonia was a result of complications due to the suppressing of his immune system to stop the body attacking Darvall's heart (Høystad, 2007).[4] Until advances in immunosuppression were made, organ transplantation procedures remained unsuccessful. The media storm that ensued after the first heart transplant was not because Louis had died. Nor indeed, whether in South Africa, the apartheid system would create a situation whereby one section of the population would become a source for another (Bound Alberti, 2010). Instead, journalists asked Louis how it felt to have a female heart or one that was not Jewish (Nathoo, 2007: 163). There were questions raised about the consequences of 'changing a soul' (Bound Alberti, 2010) because:

> for the first time one of the most important metaphors for person-hood had been cut out, handled and cleaned and then placed inside the body of another individual. In a few historic moments, the borders of one human body had been breached by the symbolic core of another.
>
> (Helman, 1991: 6)

The heart has a symbolic and cultural association with identity, affectivity, feelings and emotions. 'To have a heart to heart', to 'love someone from the bottom of my heart', 'he found it in his heart', 'to pull on your heartstrings' and 'her heart is in the right place' are all common expressions of how the heart is the emotional base of human beings, the force that is required to be humane. The symbolic heart is associated with what we know as 'being human' as emphasised by the Tin-man's plea for a heart in the *The Wizard of Oz* (1939). Indeed in *The History of the Heart* Høystad writes how the heart 'has also been made the seat of our conscience, since bad conscience is experienced as a stab or sudden pain in the heart. For that reason, the soul is placed in the heart' (Høystad, 2007: 12). The heart as a pump located in the body-as-machine has, it should be noted, an overtly strong masculine image associated with it (Emslie and Hunt, 2009), whereas the symbolic image associated with it is feminine. The heart sits awkwardly in the medical and scientific ideology of the Cartesian body-as-machine, as the 'pump or the engine for the body' while simultaneously remaining in its metaphoric space, 'symbolising the conjunction of body and soul' (Manning Stevens, 1997: 276). The heart sits uneasily in a place that views it in medical terms, like a pump or an engine in the mechanical body, but also has a symbolic and cultural association with identity, affectivity, feelings and emotions.

I'm just a broken machine?

For Louis' wife, there was an initial concern that the heart transplant had somehow changed Louis. In documentary footage shown later:

> It started with 'The Man with the Golden Hands,' which is how Louis Washkansky, chatting in Yiddish to his wife, describes Christiaan Barnard who performed the world's first heart transplant on Louis. He died a couple of weeks later … At first Louis seemed to be doing wonderfully well. She was not allowed to see him until three days after the operation … *'I was very apprehensive because I thought his personality might have changed, not realising that it is the brain that makes the person. I was happy to see he was the same Louis'*.
> ('A Knife to the Heart', BBC 1 Documentary, 31 April 1996 www.bbcactivevideoforlearning.com/1/Search. aspx?PageIndex=0&SeriesID=833, emphasis added)

Clinicians reassured her that Louis was still the same, as it was the 'brain that makes the person'. However, months before Louis' transplant, changes to personal identity through the transplantation of organs was a source of concern for the anthropologist Edward Leach in his BBC Reith Lecture address in 1967:

> The marvels of modern technology fill us with amazement but also with dread. It was alright when the surgeons just fitted us up with artificial arms and legs, but now there are people going round with plastic guts, battery-controlled hearts (pacemakers), dead man's [sic] eyes and twin brother kidneys, there begins to be a serious problem of self-identification … Am I just a machine and nothing more?
> (Quoted in Nathoo, 2007: 161)

Indeed, we can all ask 'Am I just a machine or nothing more?' If I am 'more', what kind of more is it? Descartes' (1641) view was that the body is a machine and nothing more. The 'self' therefore is one way of discussing the internal cognitive processes of an individual. In the modern Cartesian version of the relationship that a self has with its body, an analogy can be drawn between medical modifications to the body and, for example, repairs on a vehicle. The Cartesian construction of the body is one of an empty vehicle animated by the brain as the material manifestation of the self which is the driver. The vehicle, or the individual's body, is taken to a garage for repairs carried out by the 'mechanics of medical science' (Helman, 1991) if it breaks down or needs parts replaced. The medical mechanics use recycled parts (e.g. organs) separated from other body vehicles. Such modifications are mediated by the expert medical systems, that determine whose body can be repaired, replaced or possibly regenerated next, dependent on prognosis and available resources. Descartes viewed the body and the self (or mind) as two distinct and separate entities based on his 'I think therefore I am' conclusion, beginning from a starting point that his senses cannot be trusted (Farr, Price and Jewitt, 2012). In the face of the doubt that the senses can produce, Descartes considered them highly unreliable sources of knowledge. Descartes argued that the only thing that he could be sure of, the only knowledge that could be relied upon, was 'je pense, donc je suis'. The only thing he could be sure of, therefore, is 'I think therefore I am', or in the Latin, 'cogito ergo sum'. There must be, he concluded, a thinking self to be thinking. This 'I', 'who thus thought, should be something', is separate from a body that is a vehicle for the intangible, non-material substance of cognition and the self. I am just a machine, nothing more or less. Transplant surgery depends on the idea of a body that has interchangeable parts. If one of the components fail, say a kidney, then it can be removed and another inserted in its place. In this view, then, the body is like a car. Surgeons are like mechanics. The parts are exchangeable (although most do not come with a guarantee or warranty). The Cartesian idea of a split between self and body has been highly influential in the biomedical world; the body has little relation to the self and is viewed as a vessel or vehicle like a car but nothing more. Having a body – a dualistic version of embodiment – implies there are no identity or relational issues that result from making an organic addition to the body.

The brain as self

The legacy of the Cartesian ideology of having a body-as-machine, with a self that is materialised as brain and operationalised as thought, has had traction in most of the modern West, not only in that of the medical system. As Burkitt argues: '[I]n the Western world individuals have grown accustomed to a way of understanding them-selves which divides their existence between the mind and the body' (Burkitt, 1999: 7). Elevated physiologically and epistemologically, the self is housed in the brain and is the driver of the Cartesian vehicle. In modern society, the thinking self is now closely associated with the brain as the materiality of self-identity and cognition. Indeed, the 1990s was declared the 'Decade of the Brain' and neurological explanations and research from neuroscientists arguing the mind is located in the brain increasingly gained influence. Vidal, in his article 'Brainhood, Anthropological Figure of Modernity' (2009), suggests it is only in the modern era that this idea of self, materialised in the brain, became accepted wisdom. His drawing upon data and events demonstrating, for example, the decline of an Aristotelian view of the soul as the animator of the body in the 17th century and the rise and fall of the humour theory of Galen, Vidal (Vidal, 2009) demonstrates how other historical factors led to the brain-centred version of the self. Experiments showed in the 1950s that people who have epilepsy could be treated while still conscious; that split-brain experimenta-tion demonstrated how sensory information is sent to the opposite side of the brain when the two halves are separated. Along with the histological research on Einstein's brain, through to recent imaging technologies such as fMRI (Functional magnetic resonance imaging) that measures brain activity, this vast body of research showed that the search for the self, as Vidal shows, can be halted.

Then the search for the self that began with Descartes wondering 'where I am' has ended and the self is found in the brain. Localising the person in the brain – a neuro-reductionist explanation – localises the self as the mind in the brain. The second aspect of neuro-reductionism, of reducing a person to neurological matter and processes, locates 'I' identity as neurological information and cognitive function. In the neurological view of the body, the brain rules supreme in the machine and has a body that is increasingly understood in Cartesian parts (Hacking, 2007: 78).

The consequences of both the equation of self as brain and identity as neurological information is an increasing tendency to see
a self as being brain as opposed to having a brain (Vidal, 2009).
Indeed, it is an apparent fact that nowadays 'we are essentially our
brains' (Glannon, 2009: 321). It appears self-evident (pun intended)
that it is the brain where the self can be localised. Brain functioning
is clearly crucial to a being as a person, yet being a person should
not then be reduced, argues Vidal, to being a brain. However,
this is what is occurring. Mind state, consciousness and, indeed,
the thinking self is closely connected to brain state nowadays to
the extent that the two are reducible to each other. The specific
emphasis on the self as a cognitive process is also an experience
that is common to most people. When I listen to my thoughts, like
the ones I am having now when reading and writing this, I experience them as being located somewhere in my head. The philosopher
and bioethicist Leon Kass, when thinking about where 'I' am in the
body, suggested that I find my 'self' in the brain behind the eyes
somewhere:

> Science tells us the brain and no one would naturally give such an
> answer. Much of the time, I think, we feel ourselves concentrated just
> behind the eyes; When someone says 'look at me' we look at his [sic]
> face – usually the eyes, expecting there to encounter the person or at
> least his [sic] clearest self-manifestation.
>
> (Kass, 1985: 23)

It is easily assumed that the self is located in or around the head.
Terms commonly used in English language and conversation refer
to this such as 'when you need your head examined' or questioning
what was 'going on inside someone's head'. While I rewrite these
words, I can hear them in my head before, and during, the writing
of them. I have an awareness of mind and of myself thinking as well
as writing. As human beings, cognition is experientially located in
the head, and I would identify myself (or mind as the cognitive process of self) in the head area during my process of introspection,
or reflection, similar to Kass. The brain is synonymous with cognition, mind and consciousness, essentially making the brain the most
important location and site of the machine body.[5] Recent moves
to mindfulness are based on a cognitive way of reconnection: it

is a way of becoming reconnected and of 'waking up to what's happening inside of you and in the world, moment by moment' (Williams and Penman, 2014: 39).

Mrs Washkansky's concern about her husband undergoing some form of identity change through his clinical heart transplantation is assuaged when she realises that 'it is the brain that makes the person'. Her husband, after all, was the same Louis and replacing his heart had not changed him. The brain reigns supreme.

Early anthropomorphisation

In 1974, Fox and Swazey published their important book *The Courage to Fail* (Fox and Swazey, 1974) outlining the social and ethical dilemmas emerging with the new practice of clinical human organ transplantation. Indeed, this was a crucial turning point in transplant history. Although the procedure was still experimental, the effects and consequences it had had on donor families, recipients and health professionals involved, were now available to Fox and Swazey. In the United States, at the Harvard University Program on Technology and Society they had decided that organ transplant-ation was sufficiently advanced to allow them to study it in a way that was not deemed to be 'too futuristic or speculative' (Fox and Swazey, 1974: xxxiii).

In these early days, one of the issues that Fox and Swazey iden-tified is what they term an 'anthropomorphization' of the donated organ by the recipients:

> Many [recipients] still grapple with the unrequitable magnitude of the gift received and with the haunting sense that some of the psychic and social as well as the physical qualities of the donor are trans-ferred with his or her organ into their body, personhood and life.

In this early social science research, one organ transplant recipient suggests to them: 'I had a strong feeling that I had a part of another man's body; a man that I didn't even know' (1974: 31). Other research continued to marshal together accounts of how incorp-orating an organ affected the recipient's identity. Simmons, Klein and Simmons' (1987) review of several studies in the early 1970s

suggested ethnicity, youth and gender were all characteristics
thought to have been transferred from the donor:

> many investigators have described cases in which the recipient had
> difficulty incorporating the donor organ into his [sic] body image
> (Abram, 1972; Cramond 1967; Kemph 1966). Abram (1972) reports
> a case in which a white Ku Klux Klan member became active in
> the NAACP [National Association for the Advancement of Colored
> People] after receiving a kidney from a black cadaver; Viederman
> (1974) tells of a black man who fantasized that his kidney from
> a white donor was attacking him. A heart transplant patient was
> reportedly haunted by a hallucination in which the cadaver donor
> returned for her heart (Castelnuovo-Tedesco, 1973; Lunde 1969).
> Some males have felt feminized by organs from female donors
> (Castelnuovo-Tedesco, 1973; Viederman, 1974). A brother acted as
> if his masculinity was threatened when he discovered that his donor
> brother was a homosexual (Lefebvre, 1973). Viederman (1974)
> concludes that if the related donor is not liked, the kidney becomes
> a hostile 'introject' and chances for rejection are enhanced (Simmons
> et al., 1987: 67).

In this review quoted above, an incident of a biological rejection is
not caused by the recipient's immune system but through a social
rejection of the donor's organ. Years later, a similar social rejection
was experienced by Clint Hallam, who had received the world's
first single hand transplant. The hand was subsequently amputated
years later as he was said to have rejected the hand due to his
inability to accept as his own (Slatman and Widdershoven, 2010).
Attention is immediately drawn, therefore, to the importance of
incorporating another organ or limb as an accepted and legitimate
part of the recipient's identity.

Later hearts

Biomedical practices and advances in transplantation are testing
the limits of the Cartesian model of separation and duality.
More recently, research conducted by Shildrick (Shildrick, 2010,
Shildrick, 2015) suggests that very few of the 30 heart recipients
in her study were able to view the heart as a 'transferable and dis-
embodied organ that has shed all vestiges of its prior location ...

aware that their sutured bodies spoke to a different mode of being-in-the-world' (Shildrick, 2010: 18). Drawing on a 'birthing-in-reverse' analogy, Shildrick and her colleagues suggest that just as a pregnant woman needs to acclimatise to being pregnant and living with an additional self in the form of a growing baby, so an organ transplant recipient requires time to become at ease with a foreign addition; in this case an organ and not a baby. Shildrick's research suggests that nearly all of her recipients suffered a general sense of unease post heart transplant and that recipients are challenged by the 'persistence of the other' as well as the 'cultural baggage' associated with the heart insofar as it is seen as the biological and metaphorical seat of life (Shildrick, 2015). In this understanding, organs 'are always more than mere things' (Lock, 1995b), and the heart is the symbolic centre for the emotions that make human beings human. Early studies have found that some donor families donate partly due to a desire to give some form of an 'immortality' to the deceased; this is gained through allowing the donated organ to 'live on' in the recipient (Fulton, Fulton and Simmons, 1987). In one mother's words:

> I think we generally got approval from most people but kind of like, 'Isn't that nice of her to do this?' I didn't do it because I thought it was nice to do. I did it because I thought [crying], I guess, something to help him [son]. Perhaps he was alive as far as I was concerned. So his death wasn't totally a death.
>
> (Fulton, Fulton and Simmons, 1987: 352)

'Perhaps he was alive … his death wasn't totally a death' is based on a desire to make some form of life from death, a reasoning that within the recipient's body, there was a 'living on' of the person. Similarly, a donor father suggested: 'Well, it's a funny feeling. In a sense you think they're still around and yet they're not. [As long as his kidneys still function] he isn't dead down there' (Fulton, Fulton and Simmons, 1987: 352). Then for some donor families, there is a sense that organ donation is more than exchanging one body part for another.[6] Reported subjectivity alterations are not only found to be associated with organs from deceased donors. Research with living donors who donated a kidney or part of a liver show that a quarter of those participating in the study (n=111) referred to what the authors term 'identity mergers':

Recipient (brother is the donor): We joke about becoming the same person. Being myself more active than he is, he says I got the better kidney. All kinds of jokes – basically, he says, that I'm younger that he is, though I'm older, that I got the better kidney. I look younger, I'm more active.

(Simmons, Klein and Simmons, 1987: 68)

Furthermore, despite the cultural and social symbolism associated with the heart, as reviewed earlier in this chapter, it is not the only transplant that can cause the recipient to report some subjectivity alterations. Other transplantable organs such as lungs and kidney could also affect similar alterations (Sanner, 2001b). In Sharp's (1995) ethnography of 26 recipients, she suggests the integration of an organ such as a lung could result in a generic 'transformative experience'. The majority of her recipients stated that they had experienced a 'new lease of life', leading Sharp to conclude that organ transplantation is a transformative experience. One recipient of a lung transplant told her:

I wasn't myself before – you get into your own little world. I couldn't wash my hair, eat or even talk without losing my breath. My brain didn't get enough oxygen so I couldn't think straight.

(Sharp, 1995: 372)

Feeling 'stronger and younger' may be ubiquitous to any patient after a life-saving operation. It is normal, if not desirable, that patients enjoy a significant increase in their quality of life (Lock, 1995a, Lock, 1995b, Sharp, 1995). Indeed, scholars suggest that for the recipients the alleged inheritance of personal characteristics stem from an altered physical and psychological state resulting only from regaining health and of feeling better and stronger (Bound Alberti, 2010). However, recipients of organ transplantation experience negative transformations and emotions post-transplant, for example, a sense of anxiety as well as an identity crisis:

I experienced attacks of anxiety, fear of death … I ran out in the corridors totally wrecked. I couldn't find me. Who am I? Where do I come from? I was completely dizzy. It was like the familiar me but the safety I had felt was no longer there. Instead there was a new person.

(Forsberg, Bäckman and Möller, 2000: 331)

Indeed, Sharp found that 'some patients live in fear of the imagined independent or animate qualities of the new organs' (Sharp, 1995: 372).

Making the strange familiar

In the 1970s, and a practice that carries on in the UK today, authors argued that any information exchanged between donor and recipient was unnecessary and of limited benefit (Castelnuovo-Tedesco, 1973). Fox and Swazey argue that the anonymity inherent to deceased organ donation, at least in the early days, eases any guilt that the recipient and their family might have from benefiting from the donor's death (in the case of deceased donation). It also limits the recipient's knowledge of the donor's life and this, they say, 'insulates the recipient and his [sic] family from being influenced by their knowledge of the donor's person, character, social background or life history' (1974: 32). Later in 1992, Fox and Swazey continued to argue anonymity is about protecting parties 'from close encounters with the animistic, magic-infused thinking about transplanted organs in which the givers and receivers of cadaver organs often engage' (Fox and Swazey, 1992: 43). The 'animistic' thinking referred to are the narratives about how the transplanted organ is imbued with the characteristics of the donor, resulting in recipients experiencing a change from improving health as well as an alteration of self.

From the 1970s to the present day in the UK, transplant co-ordinators gate-keep the information that recipients and deceased donor families learn about each other. The UK's NHS Blood and Transplant have stated that: '[P]rotecting the anonymity of both the donor and the transplant recipient is of paramount importance.'[7] In the UK, donor families and recipients receive minimal information about each other, perhaps just age and gender, but no additional information immediately after the donation, such as ethnicity or place of donation. Letters may be exchanged after a period has passed. Eventually, and if the donor family and the recipient want to meet, this can be facilitated by a transplant co-ordinator.

To demonstrate that information about the donor is irrelevant in affecting the type of subjectivity alteration reported however, research has attempted to match the changes that are said to occur in the recipient with unknown characteristics of the donor (Pearsall, Schwartz and Russek, 2002). Pearsall, Schwartz and Russek argue that 'sensitive' transplant recipients can experience 'changes in food, music, art, sexual, recreational and career preferences, as well as specific instances of perceptions of names and sensory experiences related to donor' (Pearsall, Schwartz and Russek, 2002: 191). In the interviews they carried out with ten organ transplant recipients, as well as their friends or family members and also the donor family, despite the small number taking part in the research, Pearsall draws out the similarities in stories between the donor families and the recipients:

> Organ Recipient: If you promise you won't tell anyone my name, I'll tell you what I've not told any of my doctors. Only my wife knows. I only knew that my donor was a 34-year-old, very healthy guy. A few weeks after I got my heart, I began to have dreams. I would see a flash of light right in my face and my face gets real, real hot. It actually burns. Just before that time, I would get a glimpse of Jesus. I've had these dreams and now daydreams since: Jesus and then a flash. That's the only thing I can say is something different, other than feeling really good for the first time in my life.
>
> …
>
> Deceased Organ Donor's Wife: What really bothers me, though, is when Casey said offhandedly that the only real side effect of Ben's surgery was flashes of light in his face. That's exactly how Carl died. The bastard shot him right in the face. The last thing he must have seen was a terrible flash. They never caught the guy, but they think they know who it is. I've seen the drawing of his face. The guy has long hair, deep eyes, a beard and this real calm look. He looks sort of like some of the pictures of Jesus.
>
> (Pearsall, Schwartz and Russek, 2002: 202)

Another narrative suggests that the information that was eventually learned about the donor was contrary to the recipient's initial assumptions:

> When a 47-year-old Caucasian foundry worker received the heart of a 17-year-old African-American student, he presumed that the donor would have preferred rap music. Hence, he dismissed the idea that

his new radical change in preference for classical music could have come from the heart of the donor. However, unbeknownst to the recipient, the donor actually loved classical music and died 'hugging his violin case' on the way to his violin class.

Other stories told to Pearsall, Schwartz and Russek (2002) are about a woman who was terrified of heights until she was given the lungs of a mountain climber. Another case highlights how a seven-year-old girl had nightmares about being killed after being given the heart of a child who had been murdered. A lawyer from Milwaukee received the heart of a 14-year-old boy and inherited his craving for Snickers and a man of 25 years of age received a woman's heart and, it is reported, to his girlfriend's delight developed a liking for shopping.

How embodiment is embedded: gender in organ transplantation

In Sharp's research, a participant told her that he had received jokes from colleagues after his kidney transplant: 'You might start peeing sitting down now that you have a lady's kidney! ... So, every day I assure them, nope, I'm still peeing standing up' (kidney recipient in Sharp, 1995: 372). In her autobiography, Claire Sylvia, one of the first recipients of a heart and lung transplant in the US, remarks at length on the challenges that incorporating a new male gender posed as her health improved:

> Until the transplant, I had spent most of my adult life either in a rela-
> tionship with a man or hoping to be in one. But after the operation,
> while I still felt attracted to men, I didn't feel that same need to have
> a boyfriend. I was freer and more independent than before – as if
> I had taken on a more masculine outlook. My personality was chan-
> ging, too and becoming more masculine. I was more aggressive and
> assertive than I used to be and more confident as well. I felt tougher,
> fitter and I stopped getting colds. Even my walk became more manly
> [sic] ... A certain feminine tentativeness had fallen away. My sexual
> preferences didn't change in an overt way – I remained a confirmed
> heterosexual – but something had shifted deep within me.
>
> (Sylvia and Novack, 1997: 107)

This gendering of the organs is a finding regardless of whether the organ was from a living or deceased donor. A sister who donated to a brother is reported to have told him: 'Oh, one time I said something to him like: "If you get turned on when you walk past a man, blame it on me"' (Simmons, Klein and Simmons, 1987: 68). Interviews with organ transplant recipients conducted by Sanner showed some recipients, both male and female, welcoming male organ transplants as better and stronger as opposed to an organ from a female donor which might be considered more effeminate (2003: 394). Gender appears to be a key characteristic repeatedly brought up in stories of how organ transplantation led to a change in the recipient's subjectivity.

Cellular and pharmacological explanations

How can the characteristics of the donor, such as gender, be passed on to the recipient? Some commentators and health professionals doubt the veracity of the narrative of altered subjectivity and point to the personality effects resulting from taking immunosuppressants such as cyclosporine to dampen the immune system's response to reject the transplanted organ. It is essential that organ donor recipients take immunosuppressants to lower their immune response system, but it is also a medication known for side-effects such as developing sugar cravings. Other explanations suggest subjectivity alteration is related to the cell migration that occurs from the donor to the recipient. One of the surgical pioneers of organ transplantation argued in medical journals such as *The Lancet* that cell migration from the donor to the recipient is an essential part of the organ being accepted into the body and can be found throughout the recipient's body, with 'both the allograft and recipient become genetic composites' (Starzl et al., 1993). This idea of the recipient becoming a genetic composition of themselves and the donor is debated. The organ donor recipient will be a mix of two different types of DNA; however, it is counter-argued by some in the medical professsion that the donor DNA remains located at the site of the organ and does not circulate throughout the body. A related idea to the genetic composite one is that organs have a 'cellular memory' and that this is the cause of the subjectivity alteration experienced by the recipient. Indeed, it is one explanation offered by an organ transplant recipient:

> our bodies are made of experiences transformed into physical expression. Because experience is something we incorporate (literally, 'make into a body'), our cells have been instilled with our memories; thus, to receive someone else's cells is to receive their memories at the same time.
>
> (Chopra quoted in Sylvia and Novack, 1997: 221)

Whether cellular memory, genetic composition or pharmaceutical response, all of these explanations reside in the biomedical realm of knowledge about human bodies and are not adequately addressing why particular *social* characteristics such as gender or of music and food preferences are believed to be transferred. I will return to the idea of social contamination and fully develop it in Chapter 2.

Sociology and phenomenology

In contrast to Descartes and his body-as-machine legacy, a more complex picture emerges of the relationship between persons (inside their bodies) and their organs when exploring the recipient's experiences of subjectivity alteration post-transplantation. An alternative philosophical theory to Cartesian Dualism emphasises bodily experience as the person being their body that is involved in a perceptive relationship with the external world. This theorising can be found mainly in the work of Maurice Merleau-Ponty, who suggests that the experience of the world is both structured and limited by the body with an emphasis on perception and not Cartesian cognition. For Merleau-Ponty (1945), the relationship between the body and person is closely entwined, and is not separate but interrelated in a harmonious co-existence whereby the body is the sensory gate in and onto the physical world. The main argument in his influential work, *The Phenomenology of Perception* written in 1945, is that we are our bodies and that our experience of the world is thoroughly embodied (Merleau-Ponty, 2012). He argues that there is no other knowledge than that gained through the living body, and it is through this living of the body that 'I am my body':

> The experience of one's own body, then, is opposed to the reflective
> movement that disentangles the object from the subject and the sub-
> ject from the object, and that only gives us thought about the body
> or the body as an idea, and not the experience of the body or the
> body in reality.
>
> (Merleau-Ponty, 2012: 205)

Merleau-Ponty views the body as a way of having a presence in the
world and is, therefore, the basis of consciousness of being-in-the-
world. This 'being-in-the world' is a reversal of Descartes' 'I think
therefore I am'. 'Being-in-the-world' is 'I am, therefore I think'.
There is nothing to experience if we are not embodied. Embodiment
is experience. The focus on perception shows that interaction with
the world is an embodied experience that is meaningful and, therefore, perception is more than the physiology of seeing, for example
(Crossley, 1995). Csordas suggests 'being-in-the-world' is a term
that 'captures precisely the sense of existential immediacy ... in
a double sense: ... as a temporally/historically informed sensory
presence and engagement ... Being-in-the-world is fundamentally
conditional, and hence we must speak of "existence" and "lived
experience"' (Csordas, 1994: 10). Csordas sets the tone and lays
out the importance of the everyday experience of embodiment as
one that is culturally laden and socially located, often with a temporal and geographical location:

> If embodiment is an existential condition in which the body is the
> subjective source or intersubjective ground of experience, then
> studies under the rubric of embodiment are not 'about' the body per
> se. Instead, they are about culture and experience insofar as these
> can be understood from the standpoint of bodily being-in-the-world.
>
> (Csordas, 1994: 143)

Embodiment as a socially effected phenomenon also allows
discussions of the politics of embodiment. Following Allen-Collinson
and Hockey (2011: 332) they suggest a need for a 'sociologised'
form of phenomenology which encourages researchers to acknowledge and analyse the 'structurally, politically and ideologically-
influenced, historically-specific and socially situated nature of
human embodiment and experience' (2011: 332). For example,
Cregan shows how the ontology of embodiment (the existence of

living) and the epistemology of embodiment (of knowing) is shaped by the different social circumstances of, for example, tribalism through to post-modernism (Cregan, 2006). Feminist thinkers such as Judith Butler are concerned with how the body as gendered is constructed by societal norms over time and therefore the embodiment of social ideas around what gender is, for example, are always in process (Butler, 1993). The discussion of subjectivity alteration via organ transplantation is one that is social and culturally entrenched in ideas about embodiment of individuals as well as the embeddedness of people in relationships to each other. Anthropologists such as Sheper-Hughes and Lock produced a key text, *The Mindful Body*, in the late 1980s which also highlighted how various theoretical constructs of the body were also historically located, such as the phenomenological body, the social and the political body, and indeed the biomedical body (Sheper-Hughes and Lock, 1987). Despite this body of work on how embodiment is sociologically located (and indeed how theories of the body and embodiment are also contextually based), embodiment itself has only recently started to gain increasing recognition. In the first volume and edition of the journal *Body and Society*, Nick Crossley introduced his thinking on the difference between a sociology of the body and what he calls 'carnal sociology' or what became more widely known as embodiment (Crossley, 1995). Crossley's research draws attention to the importance of relationships with others, an 'intercorporeality'; that is, how the knowledge of a shared bodily bond which links all of us persists (1995). This intercorporeality bond that exists between humans is enriched further by Waskul and Vannini who extend it to include a 'social phenomenology' that locates 'body-self' in intersubjectivity that considers how embodiment is construed from the first-hand experience to being the same for and with, another (2006). Both intercorporeality and intersubjectivity are shown in the research of narratives from organ recipient's narratives as 'people accept that everyday their bodies are inevitably lived alongside and in response to other's bodies' (Lupton 2013: 39). Indeed, the organ donor recipient knows that the organ came from another human being and such intercorporeality is a universal feature. The human response to the organ is one that is related as a certainty based on the universal condition of being human, but simultaneously the intersubjectivity and relational element of individuals are seen in the stories told about the organs (or as Parry calls it, the 'social life': Parry, 2018).

A sociologically informed theory of embodiment based on the experience of everyday lives enhances thinking through locating embodiment in social life, structures and relationships. Subjectivity relates to an experience of embodiment that includes the body. A person's experience of their relationship with their body, a connection the word 'embodiment' denotes, is highly ambiguous. Indeed, in the social sciences, embodiment is more generally understood as referring to the flexible and transitory experiences of a person both being body and having a body (Clark, 2007, Crawford, 2014, Cregan, 2006, Crossley, 1995, Crossley, 2001, Farr et al., 2012, Featherstone and Burrows, 1995, Fielding, 1999, Haddow, 2005, Harrison, 2000, Howson, 2004, Howson and Inglis, 2001, Inglis and Howson, 2002, Lupton, 2013, Newman and Carpenter, 2013, Shilling, 2001, Shilling and Mellor, 1996, Smith, 2016, Turner, 1992, Turner, 2008, Waskul and Riet, 2002, Waskul and Vannini, 2006, Weiss, 1999). The experience of both having a body and being a body is as Evans and Lee (2002) point out:

> Our bodies serve many purposes and the ambiguity which we as human beings experience as we live in our bodies (as children, mothers, fathers, employees, patients and so on) has to be recognised…an appreciation of ambiguity is central to any understandings of our 'real' bodies
>
> (Evans and Lee, 2002: 12).

Elizabeth Grosz in her book, *Volatile Bodies: Towards a Corporeal Feminism*, argues too much emphasis is placed on the interiority of the self and not enough attention on the body. Incorporating the model of the Möbius, she argues that the advantage of restructuring our theoretical thinking away from dualisms, of mind/body or subject/object and inside/outside, is the ejection of the 'mind' as having the primary explanatory framework for identity. That is, by no longer locating the self as brain-orientated, theorists and philosophers can make more use of the body. As Grosz argues, male and female bodies are:

> incised through 'voluntary' procedures, life-styles, habits and behaviours. Make-up, stilettos, bras, hair sprays, clothing,

underclothing mark women's bodies, whether black or white, in ways in which hair styles, professional training, personal grooming, gait, posture, body building and sports mark men's.

(Grosz, 1994: 142)

A person is both experientially embodied and socially embedded and therefore subject to the same structural and relational prejudices and beliefs that living in a particular time and place has. As Evans and Lee argued in their edited book *Real Bodies* regarding race and gender:

In all cases, the social world demands that the body (male or female) meets its expectations about the physical forms of human beings. Becoming male or female is the first complex negotiation for all human beings; the nature of that resolution is then located within a particular set of expectations about race and physical appearance.

(Evans and Lee, 2002: 6)

Becoming masculinised or feminised through organ transplantation is due to how organs are believed to be the same 'sex' as the body they were procured from. In this case, gender is performative on the inside as well as the outside of the body; it is made relevant when discussing organs from men or women. The human body has an inside that retains an integrity element to it. When the skin is breached, and the viscera composition altered and changed, the consequences can also bring to the fore how far-reaching embodiment is in terms of moving inside and beyond the body, affecting and being affected by others.

Varela's account of his liver transplant demonstrates what is known as the Körper/Leib co-existence occurring in the integrity of his own body, through the process of reflection that the ambiguity is grounded within, and the implications the ambiguity of embodiment has for going beyond the individual in the case of organ transplantation:

The feeling of existence, in itself, can be characterized as having a double valence too. This is expressed as a tension between two simultaneous dimensions: embodied and decentred. Embodied: on the one hand examining experience always takes us a step closer to what seems more intimate, more pertinent, or more existentially close. There is here a link between felt quality or the possible depth of experience and the fact that in order to manifest such depth it must be addressed with a method in a sustained exploration. It is this methodological gesture which gives the impression of turning 'inwards' or 'excavating'. What it does, instead, is to bring to the fore the organism's embodiment, the inseparable doublet quality of the body as lived and as functional (natural/phenomenal; Leib/Körper). In other words, it is this double aspect that is the source of depth (the roots of embodiment go through the entire body and extend out into the large environment), as well as its intimacy (we are situated thanks to the feeling-tone and affect that places us where we are and of which the body is the place marker). Decentred: on the other hand, experience is also and at the same time permeated with alterity, with a transcendental side, that is, always and already decentred in relation to the individuality of the organism. This defies the habitual move to see mind and consciousness as inside the head/brain, instead of inseparably enfolded with the experience of others, as if the experience of a liver transplant was a private matter. This inescapable intersubjectivity (the 'team') of mental life shapes us through childhood and social life and in the transplantation, experience takes a tangible form as well. But it is also true in the organism's very embodiment, appearing as the depth of space, of the intrinsically extensible nature of its sentience, especially in exploring the lived body.

(Varela, 2001: 262)

The two perspectives (of separation and having a body versus connectedness and being a body) that make up the ambiguity of embodiment are referred to by the philosopher Husserl as the experience of the body as a 'thing' (*Körper*) or as a lived body (*Leib*) (Slatman and Widdershoven, 2010). I quote Varela at length because his reflections show that ambiguous embodiment is neither an abstract nor neutral (or even neural) static state. Varela not only dismisses the neural centric approach to subjectivity, but his decentred reference to the multiplicity of identity links the body modification via the integrity of the viscera, the subsequent subjectivity alteration and relationships with other people. That is, individuals are embodied, but as people, they are also embedded within particular social networks and temporalities. Varela's account of transplantation highlights how embodiment is being and having simultaneously, and embodiment is inevitably tied to others:

A person does not 'inhabit' a static object body but is subjectively embodied in a fluid, emergent and negotiated process of being. In this process, body, self and social interaction are interrelated to such an extent that distinctions between them are not only permeable and shifting but also actively manipulated and configured. The body (noun) is embodied (verb).

(Waskul and Riet, 2002: 488)

Absent absences, or visible absences?

Despite the discussion of how embodiment involves the relationship to others as in our intercorporeality (recognition of our biological similarity) and intersubjectivity (the recognition of social variability) it is the ambiguity of embodiment that is relevant in terms of how body modification alters our own subjectivity. It is not a question of whether embodiment is ambiguous but when this ambiguity matters. Generally, it is not a problem as our bodies are mostly absent to us. Leder, inspired by Merleau-Ponty's work but in contrast to it, generally views the body (and therefore embodiment) as a routine absence. Most of the time, our body is an absent experience. If it were a constant presence, it would simply get in the way of routine everyday living. For Leder, the body is all about absence:

> Human experience is incarnated. I receive the surrounding world through my eyes, my ears, my hands. The structure of my perceptual organs shapes that which I apprehend. And it is via bodily means that I am capable of responding ... While in one sense the body is the most abiding and inescapable presence in our lives, it is also essentially characterized by absence.
>
> (Leder, 1990: 1)

Drawing on how Leder's approach shows how everyday bodies are generally absent and how such an absence is taken for granted and little reflected upon. Fielding has argued that it is not embodiment that disappears but that it is subdued or quietened in the cognition and over-thinking that is required in daily life (Fielding, 1999). When walking, we are not thinking of the coordinated movements of the legs to work together to walk, nor the facial muscles that allow us to smile or the actions needed to extend our hand out to type these words. In the day-to-day activity, our body is absent to us (a primary absence), and it is only in times that it is challenged and tested (or its composition modified by amputation and trans-plantation) that the body becomes an absent absence; a secondary absence or dys-appearance for Leder. Leder does not draw out the implications of this fluidity between absence and dys-appearance any further nor whether dys-appearance becomes an absence. However, his argument implies embodiment is not a static state and that it fluctuates, making the ambiguity relevant when the circumstances cause an individual to reflect upon it such as the case in limb amputation and indeed organ transplantation.

Amputation and transplantation: visible and invisible absence

In dys-appearance, the body's absence in everyday life becomes very much a focal point; a 'corporeal self-consciousness' (Leder, 1990: 98). Nevertheless, what happens when parts of the body do become absent in a physical sense? That is, when a limb is amputated? How does this form of absence affect dys-appearance? Merleau-Ponty discusses the example of a 'phantom limb' when a person has undergone amputation and yet still experiences the presence of the limb; he claims that 'The phantom arm is not a representation of the arm, but rather the ambivalent presence of an arm' which is not, he argues, a cognitive assessment of the 'I think' variety, adding it as a critique towards Descartes (Merleau-Ponty, 2012: 83). Indeed, Sobchack, when giving her account of her leg amputation, highlights how the absence of her limb is an active presence (Sobchack, 2010). Demonstrating that the sub-jective experiences of amputees are important, Sobchack's account of amputation highlights how the absence of a limb is an active presence (Sobchack, 2010). Her narrative of the limb's continued presence revolves around her lived body experience:

> *where* was my leg? It had objectively disappeared in the hospital … But it had also subjectively '*dys*-appeared', its presence in absence now marked 'here' and 'there', figuring itself in odd ways against the ground of where it once had lived its ordinary form of disappear-ance, its transparent and enabling absence in presence … *looking* at my body stretched out before me as an *object*, I could see nothing *there* where my transparently absent leg had been. On the other

hand, *feeling* my body *subjectively*, ... I most certainly experienced 'something *here*' – the something sort of like my leg, but not exactly coincident with my memory of its subjective weight and length; and the 'here' somewhere in the vicinity my leg had previously occupied, but not exactly coincident.

(Sobchack, 2010: 57 emphases original)

For Sobchack, looking at her body, it is an object and yet feeling it, at the same time, is a subjective experience. Sobchack's account does not seem to dwell in the realm of proprioception as defined as that sixth sense of body awareness. The experience of embodiment for Sobchack is an absent presence, and simultaneously her reflections cause her to conclude the body is both object and subject at the same time and in the same space. Sobchack's discussion of her amputation shows how she experienced her entire body as an object, and in Leder's terms, her body was made 'asunder'.[8] Before her reflection caused by the amputation, her body is absent, and it is partly due to the reflection that, ironically, causes the duality after that. Only by focusing upon my body now am I immediately aware of it. Both Varela's account of his liver transplantation and Sobchack's of her limb amputation demonstrate how the ambiguity is 'thought into' existence and the split is created from the unity that both precedes and produces it. Gadow argues that although dualism is created by the cognition that reflects on where I am in the body, it makes the question of embodiment even more pressing:

> Let us grant for a moment that the critique succeeds in showing that the essence of human existence is embodiment, that the self is inseparable for the body ... Even when we grant this, the problem of the relation between self and body is not solved; it only becomes more interesting. Body and self, although inseparable, are not identical.
>
> (Gadow, 1980: 172)

Making the body's 'absence absent' is creating the separation between body and person that was inseparable before it. As our identity is partly generated through this introspection into our physical condition, it generates the self-knowledge regarding how it is that we are embodied. Returning to Sobchack's narration about her amputation, while the leg is no longer there, it has a presence in experiential terms, despite its undeniable physical absence.

Descartes is dead – long live Descartes!

The problem of the mind and body split born out of Cartesian Dualism is one that has been struggled with and dismissed by philosophers and sociologists who accept a dual-existence of both having and being (Ozawa-De Silva, 2002). Cartesian Dualism is not dead as it harbours within it the very connection that presupposes the duality. The connection that presupposes reflection keeps Cartesian Dualism alive. Most experience suggests the cognition is an activity that takes part in the brain. Madison argues before it is possible to treat the body as a 'thing' or an 'object' (as Descartes would have it), the body must exist, as a condition of existence. In other words, for the body to be separated from the person via reflection of the self, the person and their body are intertwined in the first instance (Madison, 1981). That a person can reflect on the nature of the self and body (as Descartes had shown), but at the same time it is the reflection that shows the separation between body and person as the body becomes an active presence. A person has to be a body in the first instance for the body to become separate to the person through, for example, reflection or focusing. Pre-reflection implies that the body is the person, and at the pre-reflexive level, we are a body and embodied (Jenkins, 2013). This is a subjective element to explore that Descartes, through his introspection, attempted to think through. He equated the result, the separation of mind and body, to the process of his reflections. Cartesian Dualism implies that there is no separation, without there being a unity, from which the separation can emerge.

Conclusion: Triad of I – identity, image and integrity

The view of the Cartesian body-as-machine is one that is argu-ably found in all areas of society and not just in the medical world. It is uncontroversial to say that in the current neuro-culture, our understanding of our bodies are that of objects. We have a body in the same way that we may own and drive a vehicle. It seems that 'I think therefore I am' is deeply rooted in Western society as it is a collective experience to feel 'I' as somehow situated in the place where cognition occurs in the brain. However, a different ideology also persists that focuses on the body as the person and is in contrast to the Cartesian Dualism that emphasises a body is a machine. The persistence of stories that transplantation, or limb loss, causes subjectivity alterations suggest a more integrated view of body and subjectivity than the medical model of the body would allow. Philosophically, phenomenologists such as Merleau-Ponty highlight how a person and the body are the same, and that 'I am' comes before 'I think'. The conditions for duality and of 'I think therefore I am' are based on a position of unification in the first place. Hence, the experience of being and having a body are simultaneously possible and are not necessarily in conflict with each other. I have argued further that this is not just a philosophical issue but a sociological one, as the modern practices of organ transplanation have thrown the ambiguity into sharp relief.

Organ transplant recipients have reported subjectivity alterations that are often associated with gender. Explaining how this can happen has involved, first, demonstrating that an organ from a human donor can contaminate the recipient with characteristics (that is, through social or cellular means or both). Second, that breaching the body boundaries is a transgression and is 'when' the ambiguity of embodiment is focused upon by the recipient. It throws up the question as to whether the person is a body or whether the person has a body. The ambiguity that was previously unimportant is no longer absent. Modifications such as an organ gain or a limb loss create a body (that has an interior as well as an image) whose 'absence' is no longer 'absent'. The experience of embodiment is brought into a 'corporeal self-consciousness' or the 'dys-appearance' as Leder describes it (1990) when a bodily modification such as transplantation or amputation occurs.

Our visible and invisible bodies are mostly absent to us; we do not focus upon our legs working in the same way that we are unaware of our heart beating or kidney's functioning. When that 'absence becomes absent' the dys-appearance makes the body's previous absence absent throwing into sharp relief how the experience of embodiment is ambiguous. This is the case whether it is an amputation or transplantation, whether the modification occurs on the inside (integrity) and out (image) and both are linked to identity.

The narratives from organ transplant recipients show that body modification to the inside of the body can cause subjectivity alterations, suggestive that the inside or the integrity of the body is vital to a person's sense of identity. Indeed, integrity has recently come to be seen as important in the area of body studies (cf. (Blackman, 2010, Shildrick, 2010, Sobchack, 2010). In Latin origins of 'integer' mean whole, complete and intact (Slatman and Widdershoven, 2010: 70) and this expresses the unity of organs within the body. This body then is part of our identity, with an integrity and image that is the 'Triad of I'. Thus, an embodiment is required that reckons on the 'outside-in' as well as the 'inside-out'. So how can the inside-out (integrity) also be outside-in (image)? This is not just an 'inside-out' experience but an 'outside-in' one. Embodiment is not just about the experience of isolated individuals, and although a person is ambiguously embodied (inside-out), people are embedded in particular environments which include relationships and interactions with others (outside-in). Organ transplantation and amputation demonstrate how porous and fluid meanings are in terms of individual embodiment that is also socially embedded when organs are taken from one individual and placed in another. There is not a static embodiment but a continual flow in the Triad of I and with others. The importance of others has to be stressed because the way that the body is configured relationally is needed. The ambiguity of embodiment becomes the focus when dys-appearance is caused by breaching the integrity of the body. Embodied individuals are embedded in social contexts, and others attach meanings to bodies, but how are other bodies that are not human constructed in diverse ways? If human recipients take on human characteristics through organ transplantation from others, would subjectivity also alter if non-human animal organs or a mechanical device are implanted? If this is the case, what more can be learned about ambiguous embodiment and the Triad of I?

Notes

1 As discussed in the introduction, I avoid using the word self. I also use subjectivity interchangeably with identity, but prefer subjectivity as it alludes to the more diffuse elements of the personal that makes it more often experiential and relational.

2 Her death in 2016 aged 49 years was said to have been caused by cancer.

3 www.theguardian.com/world/2007/oct/05/france.international? CMP=aff_1432&awc=5795_1548238741_28f7129530f66604f4ac2 0dc75ba7d3c (accessed January 2020).

4 When Louis died, the heart was removed as it was required by South African police and as Denise had died in a car accident, thus 'the heart … was an important part of two different people with separate histories' (Nathoo, 2007).

5 The ethical discussions around the Harvard Committee's decision in 1968 to redefine death as brain death coincided with the first organ heart transplant. As Peter Singer commented: 'All living things eventually die and we can generally tell when they are alive and when they are dead. Isn't the distinction between life and death so basic that what counts as dead for a human being also counts as dead for a dog, a parrot, a prawn, an oyster, an oak, or a cabbage? … Brain death is only for humans. Isn't it odd that for a human being to die requires a different concept of death from that which we apply to other living beings?' (Singer, 1994: 25).

6 Yet my own earlier research has shown that some donor families deny an immortality reason and draw parallels with replacing parts of the car and is a view of individuals' bodies that can also be found in donor family accounts of why they donated (Haddow, 2005).

7 Accessed October 2015: http://odt.nhs.uk/transplantation/recipient-coordination/donor-family-and-recipient-contact/.

8 By making the body 'asunder' suggests Leder has more in common with Descartes than might first be appreciated, for example, regarding the separation (dys-appearance) of the body and Cartesian Dualism where a separation also occurs.

2

Choosing between animal, mechanical and me?

A Czech story tells of a blind man who asked for the eyes of a young girl and was given instead, in secret substitution, the eyes of various animals. Each time, he saw what the animals saw: when he was given the eyes of fish, he saw fins and scales; when he was given the eyes of birds, he saw the sky and clouds. This story reflects the widespread folk belief that when you see with someone's else's eyes, you see what that creature sees; more broadly, when you are given someone else's organs, you take on that person's personality in some way.

(Doniger, 1995: 202)

The opening quote from the Czech folk story tells how eyes transplanted from different species have varying effects on the recipient, that is, 'eyes from birds' gave visions of the sky; 'eyes from fish' offer perspectives of the sea. As outlined in the last chapter, the reality may be as strange as it is in folk stories. Narratives have persisted since the first organ transplantation procedure conducted in the late 1960s about subjectivity alterations connected with the creation of new hybrid human bodies. It was not my intention to evaluate the claims of these organ donor recipients, but it does lead to further questions about how widespread such a contra-Cartesian belief is. The transplant recipient community is a small sample of unique individuals at the moment and perhaps only a fewer number report such alterations. As was discussed in the last chapter, the Cartesian Dualism that dominates current medical practice and thinking is one that is found more generally in society, with the modern emphasis on the brain as the materiality of self.

In this chapter, I set out to research whether embodiment is ambiguous only with the experience of body modification such as amputation or transplantation or is there a broader social-cultural belief that subjectivity might be altered when given a hypothetical scenario? To put it another way, are the narratives of those reported by some transplant recipients echoed in the expectations of those who do not have organ transplants? These are important questions because if there is any way to improve the current organ supply-demand shortage experienced almost everywhere despite alternative systems of procurement such as presumed consent, then anything that would promote the acceptability of alternative sources is an important area of exploration. Further, given the importance I stressed at the end of the last chapter on how embodiment is embedded in particular social contexts, are the different transplantable materials (human, non-human animal or mechanical) thought to have differing consequences for subjectivity?

In 2016, a series of four focus groups were carried out, followed by a representative questionnaire-based survey of young adults. The focus group study was conducted first for several reasons; mostly to explore views about the acceptability of using human, animal, or mechanical in such procedures in a deep, interactive and meaningful manner. Responses help identify and operationalise questions specifically for the survey (for example, ensuring that the option in living donation includes the word 'known'). Of course, the focus groups also generated data through the unique interaction between participants and therefore offer important data in and of itself. From 11 years to 17 years of age, 1,550 young people were then targeted in a survey. This age cohort was chosen because they are 1) possibly more open to technoscientific solutions to replace, repair or regenerate human organs given they are internet citizens and 2) least likely to perceive themselves in need and therefore offer responses unaffected by the possibility of requirement. General demographics collected in the survey were age, gender and religion as well as eating preferences, such as vegetarianism (e.g. was there a connection between vegetarianism and being against xenotransplantation?). Views could be captured by asking young people to indicate their most and least preferred options from the following:

An organ taken from a pig (a procedure known as xenotransplanation);
A mechanical device that did the work of the organ (such as implantable medical device);

A spare organ taken from someone known who was alive (that is living organ donation);
An organ grown from your cells in a laboratory (an experimental procedure known as 3-D bioprinting);
An organ taken from a stranger who has recently died (such as the current deceased organ donation system).

When given a choice between the options of animal, mechanical and human, both qualitative focus groups and quantitative data from the survey show in order of preference: a majority in favour of 3-D bioprinted ones, then followed by a preference for organs from a known individual and then a deceased stranger followed by a choice for a mechanical device, and finally, a huge majority against xenotransplantation. The popularity of 3-D bioprinting and the desire to have personalised organs relate to avoiding concerns about bodily functioning that xenotransplantation raises (reliability and compatibility), avoidable harm to others (including the animals) and knowledge about the source of the organ. Also stated in the focus groups and survey were the possibilities of becoming 'part pig'. Hence, preference was for human options and then the mechanical one. This suggests that it is important to maintain identity and integrity on two levels. First, the possibility similar to the narration from human organ transplant recipients, that pig organs can alter a person's subjectivity through the modification and breach of the integrity of the body with an organ from another (once) living being. Second, this breach is not from a human being, and therefore the boundary that separates humans from non-human animals is at risk of transgressing the categories of what is known to be human and what it is to be animal. Finally, xenotransplantation, as is the case with beliefs about possible gender alteration through organ donation, threatens an individual's subjectivity. These are all boundary disruptions that 3-D bioprinting, human organ transplantation and mechanical hearts respect. Mechanical implants such as implantable cardiac devices or pacemakers do not have the same story of other (once) living beings that organ transplantation or xenotransplantation have. Implanted devices are not contaminated by, and cannot cause contamination to the recipient by association with the once living host. I will develop the idea of contamination as a means to explain how particular social characteristics are transferred from human and indeed, non-human animals.

I turn to the practice of using non-human animal organs for therapy and transplantation in humans; a practice called xenotransplantation. Then I will outline what is currently known and achievable through implantable medical devices such as SynCardia's Total Artificial Heart device and the possibility of 3-D bioprinting. I then describe in detail the results of the focus groups and survey before concluding with a reflection on what the preferences for human, then mechanical and finally animal options tell us about the ambiguity of embodiment and the Triad of I, that is, of identity, image and integrity.

Xenotransplantation

H. G. Wells wrote *The Island of Doctor Moreau* in 1896, describing how the ship-wrecked Prendick discovers an island where non-human animals are being turned human. In a short novel written in 1915, *The Metamorphosis* by Franz Kafka, the narrative of transformation is reversed when the human protagonist awakes as a monstrous insect. There is a fascination with complete transformations from animal to human but also with different combinations of humans and animals. For example, from ancient Greek and Egypt times onwards with sphinxes (human-lion combinations), centaurs (human-horse combinations) and fauns (human-goat), to more present-day modern fictional accounts of werewolves and mermaids. Whether it is humans fully or partially morphing into non-human animals, or non-human animals turning human, these are only a few examples of what appears to be a continuing cultural enthralment with the connection humans have with animals.

Xenotransplantation turns the fiction of human and animal hybridity into a reality for medical therapy. However, skin grafts using frogs, cats, dogs, chickens, cockerels and pigs have been unsuccessful (Appel, Alwayn and Cooper, 2000), as were chimpanzee testes implanted into aged men to improve fertility (Rémy, 2014). Xenotransplantation remains an experimental procedure and has a high failure rate, as was tragically demonstrated in the 1980s when Baby Fae died after her failing heart was replaced with one from a baboon, raising questions about the ethics of the procedure, especially whether her parents gave full and informed consent (Kushner and Belliotti, 1985).

Advances in successfully creating a non-human animal and human hybrid tend to work on a much smaller scale, for example, in the conventional medical practice of using porcine or bovine material to replace human heart valves or proposals to use animal embryos for therapeutic purposes in biomedicine such as cytoplasmic embryos (Haddow et al., 2010). Success in solid organ xenotransplantation is hampered because animal organs maintain their non-human animal cellular structure, thus making them liable to attack from the recipient's immune system. The success of gene-modification such as CRISPR-Cas9 could be significant as it demonstrates how gene-editing (and immunosuppressant therapy) could potentially suppress the ability of human bodies to reject those organs not recognised as the person's own. Such a breakthrough was reported in 2016 when a genetically modified pig's heart was placed inside a baboon's abdomen, and the baboon survived for over 900 days (Mohiuddin et al., 2016). Pigs are generally preferred due to having a similar organ size to humans as well as raising fewer ethical concerns than using primates. In the UK, the Nuffield Council on Bioethics (1996) (NCoB) report on xenotransplantation emphasised that clinical trials of xenotransplantation must proceed ethically and responsibly (Fovargue, 2007) alongside the preservation of 'human dignity' (Degrazia, 2007). The report suggests that xenotransplantation practices call into question where the boundaries are between what is human and what is a non-human animal. The discourse of the value of the shared physiological features between human and non-human animals, is challenged by an awareness of the rights of non-human animals based upon a recognition that they share emotional and cognate abilities similar to human beings. This is partly why the term 'non-human animals' is used by animal activists and academics in the field of animal studies (Francione 2008).

The creation of pigs to exploit their bodies in xenotransplantation procedures is controversial when increasing emphasis is being placed on vegan and vegetarian dietary choices based on ethical, environmental and health grounds. Researchers Birke and Michael (1998) object to xenotransplantation because of the possible unethical use of animals in the xenotransplantation context:

> We might consider the suffering of humans who are chronically ill with heart or kidney disease and who face an equally chronic shortage of organs: To what extent is the possibility of alleviating

human suffering sufficient to justify raising animals in order to kill them for their organs? There is also the question of whether we consider it ethical not only to use animals for such purposes but also to deliberately create them.

(1998: 247)

Their focus group research indicates the mixing of non-human animal and human organs produces reactions of disgust or 'yuck' from members of the public (Brown, 1999, Brown and Michael, 2001, Brown and Michael, 2004, Brown, 2009). For '[Fl]esh is something about which we are culturally ambivalent, even when it comes to eating it ... [m]oving it about in the fashion of xenotransplantation is hardly likely to be culturally neutral' (Birke and Michael, 1998: 252). Similarly, Davies discusses the concept of disgust concerning xenotransplantation (Davies, 2006). This was based on focus group work with members of the public, and she focused her analysis on the 'yuck' factor, suggesting that in some cases, disgust could be a useful and instructive feeling and not one easily overcome by 'rational' scientific explanations (Davies, 2006: 432–433).

Patient experiences

Social and cultural beliefs about the acceptability of xenotransplantation are likely to vary and may be dependent on need, preference, the amount of non-human animal material used, as well as where it was going to be implanted. Although there are no successful examples of xenotransplantation, de-cellularised structures are used when repairing heart valves. Porcine and bovine tissue have been commonly used to successfully replace failing aortic heart valves since the early sixties. Porcine replacements last approximately 10 to 15 years; less in younger recipients although the reasons for the shorter life span of the valves in this cohort are not well understood. Some research with patients who have received small de-cellularised tissues instrumentally viewed the porcine implants with little evidence of concern (Lundin, 2002, Teran-Escandon et al., 2005, Idvall, 2006), although Lundin also found anxiety in her research with diabetic patients transplanted with insulin-producing porcine islet cells (Lundin, 1999). One diabetic patient who had received porcine islets reflected: 'It feels like something big and meaty. And I am wondering what way it can change me as a person. Yes, not that I'll develop a tail or anything like that – but that something will happen to me all the same' and 'Like small piglets ... tiny pig cells that I have no control over and that can pump something animal like into my body' (Eva in Lundin 2002: 337). Recipients implanted with de-cellularised porcine heart valves also demonstrated similar concerns about the transference of animal qualities (Lundin, 1999, Lundin and Widner, 2000, Lundin, 2002). A patient with Parkinson's disease reflects on the possibilities of using animal tissues in another study, suggesting that 'The personality' is in the brain. If you add a very small quantity of cells from a pig to an existing brain, that's OK. But if we are talking about replacing half of the cerebrum, then we would be replacing a large share of the individual's personality' (Lundin and Widner, 2000: 1175).

Public attitudes

A review of different acceptance rates in potential transplant patients and carers (transplant waiting/already transplanted patients; dialysis and Type 1 diabetic patients; health care professionals and members of the public/students) found an agreement to the possibility of xenotransplantation varied greatly from 80 per cent finding it acceptable, dropping to other studies finding only 19 per cent deeming it acceptable (Stadlbauer et al., 2011).

Many studies have sought to gauge public attitudes towards xenotransplantation. These are often based on attitude scales, and the results paint a relatively similar picture to each other. They show xenotransplantation can be as acceptable as human organ transplantation (80–90 per cent would accept such a procedure if necessary), but that this support drops significantly if more information about xenotransplantation is given. Or if the given scenario suggests that xenotransplantation would not be as good as a human organ transplant (Bona et al., 2004, Canova et al., 2006, Conesa et al., 2006, Lundin and Idvall, 2003, Lundin and Widner, 2000, Martinez-Alarcon et al., 2005, Rios et al., 2005, Sanner, 2006). Concerns found in this research related to disease transmission or a possible transference of genetic material, ethical issues with xenotransplantation practice, as well as fears 'about the psychological aspects of having an animal organ in the body' (Stadlbauer et al., 2011: 498). Some researchers found more favourable attitudes towards smaller amounts of non-human animal cells and tissues such as porcine heart valves rather than larger organs in the general population:

> On the one hand, an organ from an animal is larger than separate cells or tissue and might be experienced as a greater encroachment on one's body. On the other hand, it is well defined and one knows exactly where it is located, which might create a sense of security. A collection of cells is more diffuse and less well identified, but is smaller. In many situations, things that are larger are considered to be more important and could even be more threatening.
>
> (Persson et al., 2003: 76)

Lesser amounts of non-human animal organs are found to be more acceptable especially when it comes to the broader social importance placed upon the brain in terms of human identity (Stadlbauer et al., 2011). The logic presumably is that with decreasing amounts of materiality used from the source, the less likely the risk of *contaminating* the recipient. As I will discuss later in this chapter, the idea of *contamination* is a useful way to describe how using organs from a human or non-human animal donor could alter the recipient's identity. Therefore, the more materiality used to change the human body, presumably the increase in possibilities of altering subjectivity, and hence less is more. Where in the body xenotransplantation occurs affects expressed views with the brain seen as integral to the self. This highlights the social acceptability of a brain-centred approach to identity, as well as how much brain can be transplanted before the person is changed. It appears that it is not only a case of how much of the human body requires replacement but where the substitutions are made and whether it is of the same material or from a different origin.

Implanted medical devices

If there were a race to be the first to replace or repair an entire human organ, the winner would be a mechanical implant in the form of a medical device. Implantable devices (medical, aesthetic and for sensory interactions) are becoming increasingly common and complex, or 'smart' as colleagues and I have termed it (Harmon, Haddow and Gilman, 2015, Haddow, Harmon and Gilman, 2016). The number of therapeutic devices that are semi-autonomous and (partially) implanted range from cochlear and retinal implants, neuro-bionics, DBSs (deep brain stimulators), neuro-implants, vagus nerve stimulators, cardiac pacemakers, LVADs (left ventricular assist devices), artificial pancreas and ICDs. These are arguably different from prosthetics because all of these devices perform an active function rather than serving as a support structure, for example, hip joint.

In February 2012, the American-based company SynCardia reported on their website that they had implanted 1,000 Total Artificial Hearts (TAH) (www.syncardia.com/). TAHs replace the entire human heart which has to be removed and used as a bridging device until a human organ donor can be found. However, TAHs are increasingly being relied upon for long periods of time as a destination therapy, that is, when a heart transplant cannot take place. In 2015, SynCardia was approved by the United States Food and Drug Administration for this permanent use (approving it as 'destination therapy') in 19 patients who had biventricular heart failure and were ineligible for a heart transplant. The SynCardia website has numerous testimonials from patients suggesting how much the device has improved their life despite having to carry a large power supply for the TAH to be carried by or with the recipient at all times (Standing et al., 2017). Whereas this may be seen as a general inconvenience, implantable devices do pose issues about device failure, rejection and infection:

> As of 2011, 47 patients had been supported with a SynCardia TAH for greater than one year worldwide (35). The mean support time was 554 days ... Device failure occurred in 10% of patients. Systemic infections were observed in 53% of patients, driveline infections in 27% of patients, thromboembolic events in 19% of patients and hemorrhagic events in 14% of patients.
>
> (Cook et al., 2015: 2178)

Studies report individuals are aware of these risks that are associated with devices but still view them as more preferable to the problems of contamination and altered subjectivity associated with using non-human animals. In Sharp's study of 50 under-graduates, she found the majority preferred human organs, followed by mechanical devices, with none of her respondents choosing an organ from a baboon (Sharp, 2006). A few survey respondents reflected on why they would prefer a mechanical option as '[N]obody's used it before me and infected it' (Sharp, 2006: 229). One or two of Sharp's participants were worried about taking on characteristics of the baboon suggesting, '[I]f it all worked equally well, I wouldn't care. Though it would be a little strange to have a baboon heart. Would I start baring my teeth and bottom?' (Sharp 2006: 232). One survey found 77 per cent of Swedish respondents indicated more willingness to accept an organ from a relative (69 per cent), followed then by a preference for an organ from a deceased person (63 per cent), then an artificial 'organ' and the least preferred (at 40 per cent) was for a non-human animal organ. Artificial implants are viewed more favourably than using non-human animal organs by members of the public (Sanner, 1998, Sanner, 2001a, Sanner, 2001b, Sanner, 2003, Sanner, 2006). These comparative studies are important but did not include innovations such as 3-D bioprinting or identified the pig as the source of the organ (Sanner 2001b, see also Kranenburg et al., 2005).

3-D bioprinted organs

An alternative and very recent addition to proposals to repair the human body does not rely on replacement of organs from different origins such as animal or mechanical, but relies instead on the regeneration of organs: 3-D bioprinted organs from the recipient – essentially making the source and receiver the same and doing away with any middle organism. 3-D bioprinting of organs takes personalised medicine to the next level, offering the possibility of printing an individual's organs sourced from their own cells, on demand, hence avoiding contagion from other humans or non-human animals entirely. Specialised printers use biological inks (bio-inks such as differentiated-, human embryonic-, or induced pluripotent stem cells) to print layers of living materials one slice at a time, placing them on top of each other. 3-D bioprinting works with organic materials such as living cells to create structures approximating body parts from the person that needs them (Vermeulen et al., 2017). Yet, '[A]chieving the desired level of cell density, effective, vascularization and accelerated tissue maturation are remaining challenges' (Mironov, Kasyanov and Markwald, 2011). The risks of the procedure, especially using induced pluripotent stem cells (iPSCs), are unknown and have never been attempted before; such repercussions could therefore prove to be fatal (Vermeulen et al., 2017). Although 3-D bioprinting organs may one day prove to be the Promethean regeneration for the modern era, it has yet to undergo clinical trials.

Despite this lack of progress with 3-D bioprinting, it could potentially avoid the challenges that xenotransplantation raises in terms of rejection and immunosuppression as well as associated ethical concerns, in addition to possible cultural and social ambivalence about using non-human animals for this purpose. 3-D bioprinting also removes questions and concerns about the source of the organ. Would individuals prefer 3-D bioprinting despite its lack of testing and novel premise? Should it be successful, how would 3-D bioprinting compare to procedures that already make use of devices or the proposal to use non-human animal organs? Indeed, where can these options be located in terms of attitudes towards the current system of human organ transplantation, which although it cannot meet current demand, is arguably a successful procedure that is saving and improving human life?

Mixed methods: focus groups and surveys

In 2016 we carried out a series of focus groups followed by a representative survey of young people to investigate whether members of the public would prefer human, animal and mechanical as possible replacements if their organs were diseased and failing. The focus group study was conducted first for several reasons, mostly to explore questions and areas that could be discussed generally about views of biomedical technology in a deep and meaningful manner.

The focus groups were initially purposively sampled for age, religion, sporting activity and familiarity with technology hence: 1) the 65 Years of Age and Over, 2) University Competitive Fencers, 3) Computer Gamers and 4) members of a University's Islamic religion group. Although identification of group members was based on primary characteristics (such as being pre-internet citizens in the case of the 'Over 65s', or assumed technology embracers such as the 'Computer Gamers', competitive sports for individuals focused on body work, or known religious views regarding meat), the participants' identities varied by experience, demographics and interests. For example, Roy in 'The 65 Years of Age and Over' group and a 'pre-internet' citizen was a committed vegan which strongly affected his views of xenotransplantation as further discussed below. The focus group data that was generated partially informed the next phase of data collection, which was a series of questions in a survey format to young adults.[1]

Aged from 11 years to 17 years of age, 1,550 young people were targeted in a survey as: 1) possibly more open to technoscientific solutions given they are internet citizens and 2) least likely to perceive themselves in need and therefore offer responses affected by this possibility or requirement. The overall sample of young people comprised around 300 state secondary schools throughout Scotland (UK). The sampling frame was stratified by local authority, school size and urban-rural classification and a random start point ensured a representative sample of secondary schools was produced. Each school agreeing to participate in the research was randomly allocated two-year groups from S1–S6. The survey was administered by class teachers, using self-completion online questionnaires in a mixed ability class such as Personal, Health and Social Education.

General demographics were included such as age, gender and religion as well as eating preferences such as vegetarianism. The results of some of these associations between views and demographics are reported below. The questions were generated partly from the focus group data as well as in close collaboration with Ipsos MORI, who are a large UK market research company commissioned to carry out the study (www.ipsos.com/ipsos-mori/en-uk).

I expected that posing questions about abstract ideas of identity and subjectivity of other humans as well as other species would be extremely difficult for participants to engage with or respond to. The focus groups were difficult to recruit partly due to this reason. Informal feedback suggested that this was partly based on a perceived lack of qualification by those approached to discuss the topic of animal, human and mechanical technologies. Indeed, in the focus groups, I felt I spent too much time explaining the benefits and risks of the technologies, which restricted further opportunities for their contribution. Apart from the initial choice question that was given to survey recipients, no additional explanation was offered during the administration of the survey about the different human, animal and mechanical. Posing questions about hypothetical future technologies is both conjectural (preferences for using human or non-human animal technologies that do not exist) and rhetorical (even if they did exist the decision whether someone would receive one would be clinically informed and not based solely on individual choice). The methodological context is hampered by the creation of a question format of a 'what if' variety ('what if this happened'). The difficulty in answering the questions is demonstrated with a large proportion of young adults suggesting that they 'Don't know' or 'Prefer not to say' (26 per cent) indicating a lack of respondent confidence in how to respond when limited information is offered. This is bound to be the case when some participants were very young, for example, only 11 years old. Survey respondents were therefore encouraged to give additional open comments at the end of the questionnaire explaining their choice, even if it was a 'don't know'. Although it is not possible to link these comments made in the open section of the survey to actual respondents (as the respondents and responses were irreversibly anonymised), the comments left in the open section offer extremely rich data; the frequency of comments was numerically counted and similarity noted (e.g. 'It's a pig' was a very common response). The survey was analysed with the use of SPSS v11.5 and the open comments imported into an Excel spreadsheet. The findings below therefore draw on all data from the survey results in the questionnaire, the frequency and content of the open comments and the focus group discussions.

Results: all the humans (3-D, living and deceased)

The following key question was offered in the survey:

Sometimes people's organs (e.g. their heart or their liver) can stop working properly. If this happens, they need to have that organ replaced. Imagine you needed to have an organ replaced because it wasn't working properly, how would you want it replaced? Please rank the following options from 1 to 5 in order of preference (1 being the option you most prefer and 5 being the option you least prefer).

The following options and short explanations were given and rotated in different order in the survey:

- An organ taken from a pig (a statement to describe xenotransplantation);
- A mechanical device that did the work of the organ (to refer to implantable medical devices);
- A spare organ taken from someone you knew who was alive (to avoid confusion it was stated that this was a related living organ donation and with an organ that wasn't needed, hence 'spare');
- An organ grown from your own cells in a laboratory (3-D bioprinting);
- An organ taken from a stranger who has recently died (the current UK system largely based on deceased organ donation).

Despite my earlier misgivings about the difficulties participating in the study would cause, the overall findings were unequivocal. All the human organ options (3-D bioprinting, living donation and deceased donation) were the favoured options with 3-D bioprinting by far the most preferred (21 per cent or 22 per cent) (as shown in Table 2.1):

Table 2.1 How would you *most* want the organ replaced?

	Frequency	Per cent
An organ taken from a pig	25	**1.6**
A mechanical device that did the work of the organ	123	7.9
An organ taken from a stranger who has recently died	179	11.5
A spare organ taken from someone you knew who was alive	336	21.7
An organ grown from your own cells in a laboratory	345	**22.3**
Don't know	407	26.3
Prefer not to say	135	8.7
Total	1550	100.0

The 'Computer Gamers', 'University's Islamic' group and the '65 Years of Age and Over' groups stated their top preference would be for 3-D bioprinted organs, thus confirming an overall preference in the results, for an organ to be created from one's own body. As Sophia in the 'Over 65s' group suggests:

> I would prefer to have something that is connected in some way to a human being either past or present or manufactured from something in the ... Well, just having a connection to a human in some way, even it was made from cells cultured in the lab originally, an imaginary source.

Statements in the open part of the survey supporting 3-D bioprinting ranged from 'They [organs] come from me', being from 'my own cells', 'it was your own', 'part of my body', 'part of me', 'my own cells in my own life' and that this was preferred from other human bodies, as it was from 'my own body and not from someone else'. However, Adila, in the 'University's Islamic' group pointed out that should 3-D bioprinting become a possibility in the future, potentially avoiding issues around rejection (as is the case, for example, with human transplantation and xenotransplantation), this would be an expensive first world option:

> I think I would, of course, prefer my own stem cell and my reason is like what I pointed out earlier. Sometimes our body rejects a new organ, someone else's stem cell might have a different reaction, there is a risk, the issue of risk. However, going back to the initial stem cells in, yes, I would prefer that, but on the other hand I think it's quite an exclusive option because there are many countries, we cannot afford such technology, and we have to depend on a human donor, so it's great, but it's very limited in how it reaches up to people and there are a lot of people who are in need of organs, and probably people from first world country could develop this technology. The only thing your own stem cells do for organs that can be in turn donated to people who cannot afford it in third world countries, I think that's a great option, yeah.

(Adila)

The human living options were stated as being the preferred option, although deceased organ donation (n=179) was the least popular of all the human options. One reason for ambivalence about deceased organ donation was that the deceased donor was a stranger: 'I don't know the person or how they lived their life', 'because it seems risky and I wouldn't know their past'. The other reason for dislike was that the donated organs came from an individual who had died and 'because they are dead and that's weird', 'I don't like the thought of someone's dead organs in me; they wouldn't work'. Those who supported deceased donation did so for the same reason that those against it gave; it was 'because the person was dead' and the 'organs would not go to waste'.

Organs from deceased donors appear more disliked by young men (38 per cent; n=109) than young women (61 per cent; n=69) in the current sample. Why young male respondents were more likely to dislike the current way that organs are procured from deceased donors is unclear and could not be ascertained from this data. The next best substitute would be of a known living individual; the quality of being known seems almost as important as being human. A reason for not favouring the current deceased procurement system, in light of these future possibilities, is because the donor is both deceased and a stranger. So, to summarise, an organ created from the individual is preferred, a known organ donor is liked, but a deceased stranger's organ will do. What will not do, however, is using organs from a pig, as I turn to next.

Never xenotransplantation

I have emphasised in previous chapters that the materials that are placed inside the body are also ones that are socially and culturally embedded, and this would most obviously be the case when it comes to views around the use of animals for transplantation. 3-D bioprinting, for example, potentially avoids ethical, practical, religious and social challenges posed by xenotransplantation (Brown and Michael, 1998). The survey results (shown above in Table 2.1) demonstrate less than 2 per cent of the young adults (n=25) gave xenotransplantation as their preferred option. It was said by a few individuals in the focus groups to be very similar to consuming meat. In the 'Computer Gamers' focus group, the following exchange occurred between Chris, Oliver and Timothy:

> **Chris:** Does it make a difference if you can use the rest of the pig for meat?

Oliver: That makes it better. That makes it better.
Chris: What's that again, what's that kind of meat? Sorry.
Oliver: If you get a heart for a transplant ...
Timothy: And, bacon.
Oliver: ... then you also get bacon, so ...
Chris: To ruin the heart that you just got.
Timothy: To be fed to the person that's got the heart.

Apart from the apparent jocular nature of the exchange between the male focus group participants, a view is expressed that if a person consumes meat then this should make the person hold positive opinions about using animals for xenotransplantation. In the '65 Years of Age and Over' focus group, Roy who was a life-long vegan expressed a similar view in a far less humorous tone in an exchange with Cameron (who consumed meat):

Roy: I'm a 30 years vegan, so it's quite clear my decision on that, I think it's an appalling idea. I think it is again the exploitation of animals and whatever which I think, don't think we really should be involved in ...
Cameron: Not enthusiastic.
Roy: We agree, yes, we have found common ground probably for totally different reasons.
Cameron: Given that I enjoy a bacon sandwich, I think it would be illogical for me to say I wouldn't take something from a pig, again providing that it is done without cruelty.
Roy: ...if you're prepared to put it down your throat, then why wouldn't you be prepared to put it in your leg or whatever, your heart?

The challenge from Roy is that those who consume meat should be in favour of xenotransplantation as 'if you're prepared to put it down your throat, then why wouldn't you be prepared to put it in your leg or whatever, your heart?' The survey results paint a different story, however. Roughly equal numbers of those who self-identified as vegetarians (46 per cent) and those who consumed meat (48 per cent) said they were against xenotransplantation. It may be that the practice of transplanting pigs' organs is not equivalent to choosing to consume pork or ham. Through the digestive process, meat consumption will leave the body, whereas xenotransplantation will not and would be a permanent addition. Neither does eating meat instigate a rejection process by the body, whereas a xenotransplanted organ does. In the 'Competitive Fencers Group', Amy discussed the issue of immunosuppression required for the recipient's body so as not to attack a non-human animal organ:

> Amy: If it was a last resort I would definitely accept an animal organ. But I would accept a human organ over an animal organ if they were both available. Because even if it was like perfectly functional, the same, but there are risks associated with animals because they are different, physiologically. So, if you get down to like cellular level with all the receptors and everything, it means you have to be on ... I know you have to be on immunosuppressants in a human, but you have to be on more, I think, with an animal.

Such discussions echo the challenges of over-riding the body's immune response to attack any organic materiality that is foreign to the recipient's body.

If lifestyle decisions about meat consumption appear to have little relationship to xenotransplantation, does religious instruction forbidding eating meat play a role in being against xenotransplant-ation? Some authors have suggested it is acceptable for religions against eating meat, for example those who identify as Muslim, to accept pigs as organ substitutes (Welin and Sandrin, 2006, although see also MacKellar and Albert Jones, 2012) despite instruction that says otherwise. Fifteen of the 27 respondents who self-identified as Muslim in this survey were not in favour of using pig organs for xenotransplantation. Some participants chose to identify them-selves as Muslim in the open comments section, saying that because the pig was not halal, it was an 'unclean' animal. In the following exchange, which occurred in the 'University's Islamic' group between Azzam and Leilah, Azzam is trying to articulate why pork consumption is unacceptable:

> Azzam: For example, like pigs are seen in Islam as ... so if you look like ... I'm trying to say ... like for example, pigs and stuff, like they also like ... the reason why they don't ... I think the reason is because pigs are like ... they play around in mud and stuff.
>
> Leilah: Lay there in faecal matter.
>
> Azzam: And they also eat their ...
>
> Leilah: Faecal.

Azzam: Yes and their own poo, so they're generally seen …
I was thinking of a way not to say that, by the way, if you
didn't get it. So yeah.

Importantly, the association of pigs with dirt was articulated
regardless of religious affiliation. The frequency of the comments
(such as, 'It's yuck, disgusting, gross, unclean', 'It's a farm animal
with a very unhealthy diet' and pigs are 'disgusting, rank, not natural, grim, vile, rank') outnumbered any explicit or implicit link to
religious affiliation. Not only was the pig thought dirty, but it could
also be a vehicle for diseases: 'the pig could have had a disease',
'because pigs are disease-ridden creatures', 'pigs can have some
nasty diseases'.

Other comments were made that were not as clearly articulated
such as 'It just feels strange' and 'It doesn't sound right', 'it would
especially make me feel mentally uncomfortable', 'it would creep
me out', 'it's not nice to think about', 'I don't want a pig/animal
inside me'. Having a pig's organ would make someone 'part pig'
and that the risk of using non-human animal organs was not just
about practical or ethical questions but had to do with personal
identity issues. Comments included: 'I would hate to have an organ
from an animal, I wouldn't feel right having a pig's organ', 'I don't
wanna be part pig, cos I would be pig', 'I don't want a pig inside
me', 'I would feel awkward about having a pig organ'. Very often
the reason given in the survey's comments section for being against
xenotransplantation was stated matter-of-factly: 'It's a pig'. This
exact phrase occurred frequently suggesting a shared understanding
of the reason that pigs would not be acceptable did not require any
further elaboration.

Yuck!

Responses in the current research suggest the pig for use in xenotransplantation is dirty, physiologically incompatible and potentially a vehicle of disease. Previous studies show that proposals
to mix non-human animal and human organs produces public
reactions of disgust or 'yuck' (Brown, 1999, 2009, Brown and
Michael, 2001, Brown and Michael, 2004). Kass (2002) relates

'yuck' to a 'wisdom of repugnance' that is not just a matter of individual taste but is a powerful way to discuss how reactions to the way that such proposals are challenging what is considered as 'natural':

> The contemporary need for naturalness can be better understood as a response to the fact that technology makes reality more and more makeable and, consequently, more contingent. Advancing technology changes everything that is, into our object of choice ... [I]f human nature itself becomes makeable, it can no longer naively be laid down as the norm.
>
> (Swierstra, van Est and Boenink, 2009: 274)

The Nuffield Council on Bioethics' (2015) more recent analysis of the role that the concept of 'natural' plays in public debate concluded that it is a term to be avoided, mainly because of the variability of the way it is used. There may be a stable interpellation between classifications of what is natural that only arise when it is challenged – challenging the perceived boundaries of the natural illuminate where the edges of the natural are.

'Yuck' echoes anthropologist Mary Douglas' arguments about challenges to the boundaries between species and is linked to ideas about 'Pollution behaviour' which is 'the reaction which condemns any object or idea likely to confuse or contradict cherished classifications' as out-of-place (Douglas, 1966: 36). Pollution behaviour is invoked when controversial crossing and blurring of boundaries between bodies and species occurs. Although pigs, or any other non-human animal for that matter, may not necessarily be considered unclean (although pigs are considered unclean by some because of scavenging faeces and dirt as discussed above), their usage in transplanting human bodies challenges the known schemata of what it is to be a 'pig' and what it is to be 'human'. Indeed, Douglas suggests that the pig is the 'odium of multiple pollution' (Douglas, 1972: 79). Pigs are entities that transgress familiar and taken-for-granted boundaries between species (Chakrabarty, 2003, Alter, 2007, Robert and Baylis, 2003). The creation of chimaeras and hybrids, for example, is seen as 'an affront to the hierarchical superiority and separateness of the human species' despite the practice of breeding animals and hybridised plants (Knoppers and Joly, 2007: 284). Views about xenotransplantation might be therefore closer to understandings about chimaeras and the mixed bodies of species, rather than vegetarianism. As I have shown, there is little variation in terms of religion or vegetarianism beliefs that helps explain respondents' negative views of xenotransplantation. Rather, the finding from this research suggests a deeper-seated repugnance expressed as 'yuck' due to the perceived challenge to what is considered the natural species' boundaries. One last comment worth mentioning is that not everyone thought that pigs' organs would affect identity. As Adila suggests: 'I don't think it affects me as a person. I think it ... if I needed, it's urgent, I might die without it, I think I would take it and it will not affect me as a person, I'm really sure of it. Neither my cognitive ability, my spirituality, my emotions, so ...'. This was not a common response, but it does highlight that a person's need for an organ, even an animal's one in the case of xenotransplantation, may overcome any social or cultural ambivalence or abhorrence about the source.

So, what about machines?

Overall, data in this research suggest using devices to replace whole organs was not as popular as human organs. However, they were not found to be as unpopular as using animal organs. Azzam and Adila in the 'University's Islamic' group exchanged views around the difference between an artificial device and an organic living thing, with Adila stating that she would prefer the human option as it retains the necessary 'human element':

> **Azzam:** And also the system, it's a man-made thing, as in it's not exactly ... I say manmade ... I mean, I think I would rather use that, yeah.
>
> **Gill:** Can I push you a little bit more on the distinction between it being artificial, say, manmade, we'll go with manmade, that's fine, it's okay and animal, is there something ...
>
> **Azzam:** Well, I mean, there is obviously a difference because it is not a living creature. I don't want to go all hippy and try and like ...
>
> **Gill:** No, no ...
>
> **Azzam:** But obviously it is different, it's a completely different thing because it's not a living thing, it's not something that

God has created, it's just something … it's not a man creation, but it's not real, it's not that valuable.

Adila: Quite the opposite, actually, I wouldn't take it (machine). I would put it last (in terms of preference), simply because I think the human connection is very important. Taking an organ from a human donor to me, is the best option. I know it sounds macabre, but because I myself, I have … expressed earlier, when I die I would like to strip myself bare in the sense that you take everything I have for use of someone who really needs it and I think on that note I would prefer to take from human being who is obviously deceased, but it's not that I undermined the competency or the value of machines, but it's just that taking something human is essentially human of me. It's more sentimental, there's nothing … I have no scientific or religious opinion on this, it's just sentimental.

In this exchange, Adila and Azzam agree on the value of the human body. But Azzam suggests because a machine is less valuable then the machine should be used, whereas for Adila because the human is more valuable than a machine, the human is preferred. Other reasons for not wanting to have a machine used for the repair of the human body, were generally similar to the following: 'you'd feel like a robot or a freak', 'makes me less human', 'because I don't want a machine inside my body', 'I don't want to be cyborg', 'I don't want metal inside me'.

The small number which indicated the mechanical implant was their most favoured option referred to popular films, suggesting that 'I want to be like Iron Man or the Terminator', and 'It would be cool being part-robot', 'It would be cool to be Robocop', 'I feel that it's easier and I'd be more comfortable with that than someone else's organ in my body'. Other survey respondents suggested that, due to thorough testing and advances, technology was felt to be 'smart': 'Because technology now is really smart so I would feel safe having something smart doing the work.'

One or two individuals in the focus group took a more pragmatic approach, choosing to focus on the stable functioning of the implant over-riding any preferences for materiality (whether human, animal or mechanical). Daniel, in the 'Computer Gamers' focus group, was consistent about this, repeating that, 'Not really, *as long as it works*, I keep saying this, I know' (Daniel, 'Computer

Gamers' focus group, emphasis added). Technological vulnerability is an issue raised by survey respondents and those in the
focus groups. Fears about technology breaking and malfunctioning
were routinely expressed. Biohacking was only mentioned in the
'Computer Gamers' focus group, however:

> **Timothy:** Well, I think my point was the same technology that
> could be used to control the misfiring of epilepsy could be
> used in other ways that aren't quite as seemly ...
>
> **Elizabeth:** Also, to murder people potentially just find the right
> frequency and you fry your brain or stop your heart.

Machines do break, rust and malfunction. These concerns about
the reliability of technology, including functionality and malicious
hacking, are issues are returned to in the following chapters when
I discuss the becoming of an everyday cyborg.

Contamination and brains

Unexpectedly, in the 'Computer Gamers' focus group, conversations
included allusions of equating the human body to a car, and
inserting devices then makes the human body a 'changed vehicle'
echoing the Cartesian Dualist view of the body-as-machine, or as a
car or other vehicle:

> **Timothy:** I'm just thinking of an old 'Star Trek' episode, because
> ... oh, no it was one of the films actually, 'Data' the android
> talking to a kid and he's talking about how he doesn't know
> what it's like to grow up because the kid is constantly in flux,
> he's growing all the time and he [Data] doesn't have that. So,
> like if you were to suddenly be in someone else's body, you
> would have totally different size of arms, totally different
> size of legs, how long would that take you to get used to?
> A changed vehicle.
>
> **Chris:** I suppose it's a much more convoluted than like buying a
> new car type of thing.

In this group, discussions about mechanical implants led to talk
about the consequences it would have for the human body and subjectivity. Oliver and Elizabeth (in the exchange below) consider

how much of the body could be replaced before a 'cyborg' identity would be created:

> **Oliver:** I suppose there's going to be reasonable gap between people getting them and then people also getting enough of them that you can say they are almost completely cyborg.
>
> **Elizabeth:** Yes, so pretty much we can change everything, you can just be a cyborg.
>
> **Gill:** Everything?
>
> **Elizabeth:** As long as your brain is there it's still you.

Elizabeth's statement, '[A]s long as your brain is there it's still you', is reflective of the modern idea of the self, that is, materialised in the brain, with cognition as the key process of selfhood. It echoes the widespread belief held in contemporary society that the mind or self is closely associated with the brain as the materiality of self-identity and thinking as cognition (Vidal, 2009). It echoes the statements made to the wife of Louis Washkansky, the first person to receive a heart transplant, that it is not the heart that is the loci of personhood, but the brain. This discussion also echoes the philosophical question mentioned throughout this book about 'The Ship of Theseus' and how much of a ship needs to be replaced before it is no longer the same ship. In discussions of replacing human bodies, the experiment can be stated, as it was in these focus groups: 'How much of a human being has to be replaced before that person is no longer the person they once were?' Williams argues that in creating the cyborg it is 'best conceptualised on a continuum with the human organism at one end (i.e. the "all-human pole") and the pure machine (automaton) or artificial intelligence (AI) device at the other' (Featherstone and Burrows, cited in Williams, 1997: 104). This depends on a Cartesian 'body-as-machine' (discussed in Chapter 1). Bodies are a quantitative sum of body parts, which are altered through the addition and subtraction of materiality and not by any differences in the type nor kind. In the '65 Years of Age and Over' focus group, similar discussions took place about 'where the person was' when replacing body parts; either materialised as the brain or in the heart:

> **Jacob:** Well, you have the question of head transplant and which is getting transplanted, the head or the body? So, as far

as I can see at the moment the head is the important bit, but in the future, we might discover it's a minute part of the head that's important.

Roy: So, that sort of person, so if Jacob and I swapped over, right, Jacob would become me with my marvellous body and I would get stuck with him. That's as far as we know for now.

Cameron: But, there are some cultures that put great emphasis on the heart and a lot of people believe that, but as far as we can tell at the moment it is the head.

Gill: What do you all think?

Sophia: You could still have a mechanical body with a brain operating everything.

Discussions show that almost everything in the human body can be replaced with mechanical parts apart from the person's brain. This stands in contrast with beliefs about xenotransplantation when 'less is more', and not even fractional parts of the human body can be replaced with pig's organs. No one in this research (or indeed in the others I reviewed earlier on in this chapter) raise the consequences of replacing all of the human body apart from the brain with non-human animal parts. The idea that large parts of the human body could be replaced with non-human animal organs never arose and is notable for its absence. It would appear that the cultural fascination that is held with non-human animal and human hybrids is not shared with the desire for creating them. The social scientist Sanner proposes the concept of *contamination* as a way of offering a social explanation to address how these characteristics from non-human animals such as pigs could be transferred (Sanner, 2001a, Sanner, 2001b):

> This law [contagion] states that things that have been in contact with each other or have belonged together may influence each other through transfer of some of their properties via an 'essence'. Such a contamination remains after the physical contact has ceased and may be permanent. The rule is 'once in contact, always in contact'.
>
> (Sanner 2001a: 1497)

Organic materials can *contaminate* the recipient with pig-like characteristics, as Sanner suggests: 'once in contact, always in contact'. It is unsurprising to find that those members of the public asked about how they might feel about xenotransplantation and using pig organs were worried giving them pig organs would also give them pig characteristics; making them more pig-like. 'In essence, when organs are made of flesh and blood, recipients find it impossible to forget where they came from' (Sharp, 2006: 240). The idea of contamination (Sanner 2001a) can be applied to human organ transplantation to explain why human organs can carry within them the social features of the human donor as was discussed in Chapter 1. Although cellular and pharmacological explanations have been put forward by some commentators, there are additional factors to consider about not only why the organs are thought to be able to transmit characteristics, but also how social characteristics such as gender transferred.

Other researchers discuss contamination as the 'acquisition of possessions of another person that have been intimately associated with that other person' (Belk, 1987: 151). Wearing someone else's underwear, eating pre-chewed food and using another person's toothbrush, in Western society, are all examples of an association with another person that may make some individuals feel unsettled (Belk, 1987). For some, as in used underwear, this intimacy has the opposite effect of unease or even disgust, and the contamination can be a desired fetish and commodity by some. The social porosity and contamination that materials have, 'once in contact, always in contact', applies to organic fleshy beings, and not technological devices when implanted into bodies. In the next chapter, I discuss why this is the case and what are the implications for identity living as a techno-organic hybrid.

Conclusion: organ rejection and contagion versus technological infection and invasion

The most popular option to replace failing organs in the human body found in this research was for 3-D bioprinted organs grown in a laboratory from an individual's cellular material; this clear preference was made. Ideally, 3-D bioprinting organs avoided subjectivity alterations caused by organs from *any* other organic sources. By keeping the materiality of the donor and recipient the same, there was no better way to avoid the possibility of changing who you are by altering what you are. The popularity of receiving organs from someone you know or ones that are 3-D bioprinted in the current study relates to avoiding concerns about bodily functioning as is found in using mechanical devices (e.g. reliability and infection), avoidable harm to others as could be produced through xenotransplantation or living organ donation and perhaps avoiding knowledge about the 'dirty' origins of the organ from a pig.

Preference for 3-D bioprinting was followed by a stated desire for an organ donated by a known living donor. If a personalised printed organ is the most highly valued because it comes from the recipient; then the next closest to this option socially and physically is a preference for an organic living human source, known to the recipient. As living donation is often conducted in the UK between two individuals who are related, this choice suggests that when a participant cannot have an organ identical to them in identity terms (a 3-D bioprinted one), then an organ 'known to be as close to me' as possible is a narrative for this selected option. Knowledge of the donor appeared important to some respondents and something that was not generally possible in receiving a transplant from a deceased stranger (although social contact can be made via the transplant co-ordinator as discussed earlier). Knowing the story of the organ from another human body highlights a preference not to cross the species boundaries generally or disrupt the embodiment of the individual specifically.

I argued that Sanner's (2001a) theory of 'contamination' was an important reference point to think about how meanings attached to organic material are porous and transcend biological boundaries between bodies. Xenotransplantation and human organ donation, therefore, are able through contamination processes to modify the recipient's body and alter subjectivity. Xenotransplantation was almost universally disliked and created a range of concerns about the ethics of using animals in such a way and physiological incompatibility with human bodies, for example. Some comments were made about whether xenotransplantation would make the recipient 'pig-like'. This produces yuck-type responses concerning the ontology of what a non-human animal is. The identity crisis relates to the distinction between humans and non-human animals, and concern about the boundaries of either are not crossed. Of such attempts at xenotransplantation, the feminist technoscience scholar Donna Haraway writes of the 'ethical perplexity – for animal rights activists as much as for the guardians of human purity' (Haraway,

1999, cited in Kirkup et al., 1999: 165). The porosity of the contamination that can result from mixing humans' *inter-species* shows
the possibilities of *intra-species* boundary disruption between non-
human and human and why the natural boundaries that separate
the species require observation and surveillance.

Technoscientific advances in biomedicine, such as xenotransplantation, challenge what is human identity and therefore can be
expected to produce 'yuck'-type responses in relation to the ontology
of what a non-human animal is – as a threat to species identity (on
the abstract level). But 'yuck' is also apparent on challenges being
made to the individual's body and identity changing what she is;
altering who she is. No matter how close the biological similarity
between humans and other species is, as espoused by clinical and
medical researchers attempting to alleviate the human organ donor
shortage, it does not follow that there is a positive socio-cultural
acceptance from sharing visceral spaces between humans and
animals. In sum, therefore, there is a preference for human organ
replacements to be sourced from the same or related (person), and
although similar (other human bodies) might do, different (non-
human animals) will not.

Note

1 The focus group discussions took place in a mutually agreeable location generally lasting an hour and a half. Discussion began with
   exploring ideas about the relationship an individual has with the
   body and was followed by a wide-ranging conversation about human
   organ transplantation, willingness to accept a xenotransplant, as well
   as novel technologies such as 3-D bioprinting. In the focus groups
   permission was sought to record and reassurances about confidenti-
   ality given (a mixture of first names and pseudonyms are widely used
   in the following accounts). Focus groups were transcribed verbatim
   and the text imported into a computer aided qualitative data analysis package aiding the management of data (Nvivo 11). A constant
   comparative method generating codes from the data, and themes from
   the inter-relations between codes was used and is an approach loosely
   informed by Grounded Theory. However, a more abductive approach
   to thematic generation was taken overall, that is, with a knowledge of
   previous research and a sensitivity that new and unanticipated data
   would emerge (Blaikie, 2007).

3

Reclaiming the cyborg

Introduction

Previously in Chapter 2, research findings from those who took part in the survey and focus groups demonstrated that if people were made to choose between human, animal and mechanical materials as possible medical therapies, there was a clear preference expressed for regenerated or transplanted human options, followed by implantable medical devices, which were in turn preferred over xenotransplantation.

By drawing on Sanner's (2001a) theory of contamination, mechanical implants do not have the same properties of contamination from the other (once) living beings, as I concluded in the previous chapter. Implanting devices avoids the subjectivity alterations that organic parts may cause the recipient. Mechanical parts have no association with the once living and are not contaminated by them, and cannot in turn, therefore, contaminate the recipient. Whereas organ transplants can cause episodes of rejection, implantable devices are associated with malfunction and infection. In this chapter and the following Chapter 4, I take a closer look at the issues that inserting machines into the body can cause their recipients.

Implanted medical devices are relied upon by medical professionals and patients alike, offering the possibilities of an increase in the length and quality of lives. While a broad understanding of the term 'implantable' might include those technologies that are consumed (e.g. pharmaceuticals), such products are not intended to be permanently incorporated as an active medical device which is placed inside the body. An active medical device is an instrument, which, with its software, can be used for diagnostic and therapeutic purposes, relying on a power source other than that generated by the body. The Active Implantable Medical Devices Directive (1993) (AIMD 90/385/EEC as amended by 2007/47/EC) defines an active medical implant as:

> any active medical device which is intended to be totally or partially introduced, surgically or medically, in to the human body or by medical intervention in to a natural orifice and which is intended to remain after the procedure.

Implantable medical technologies that augment and replace human organs have become smaller, cheaper and even 'smarter' in the last 40 years or so. Implantable medical technologies such as CIs and glucose monitors, cardiac devices such as ventricular assist devices, pacemakers or ICDs and DBSs are examples of medical technologies that are becoming increasingly 'smart' (Haddow, Harmon and Gilman, 2016). As colleagues and I have noted elsewhere, these devices are smart because they are capable of being responsive to changes within the body they were implanted in without human intervention (Harmon, Haddow and Gilman, 2015). Such medical implants are more sensitive, responsive and autonomous in their functionality when compared to the static and stationary hip or knee joints, artificial skin and implanted corneas.

ICDs and life with a heart device

The human heart can be viewed as a pump or engine in the Cartesian body-as-machine and can be bypassed, stented, transplanted, beta-blocked, ablated, paced and replaced and, importantly, defibrillated by implantable cardiac devices (ICDs). ICDs are one of the increasingly 'intelligent' implanted technologies playing an accepted 'normalised role' in peoples' lives, that is, as colleagues and I have suggested elsewhere they are on the path to becoming mundane, everyday and ubiquitous (Harmon, Haddow and Gilman, 2015, Haddow, Harmon and Gilman, 2016). We have argued that implantable technologies are 'smart':

> Indeed, our lives are increasingly enacted within an intricate web of increasingly 'smart' technologies, which are not just performing *for*

us, but also *on* us and *within* us. By 'smart', we mean they exhibit one or more of computational intelligence, autonomous operation and responsiveness to environmental changes (i.e. they monitor, transmit, and potentially initiate a treatment action).

(2015: 231)

ICDs demonstrate more than one of the categories we proposed of autonomy, intelligence and responsiveness. Autonomy includes Wiener's classic definition of 'cybernetics', from the Greek word 'kybernutos' meaning 'governor' of a system (Wiener, 1961). ICDs also have features of an autonomous feedback mechanism operating as a closed-loop system, elements that, I go on to show, are stressed by Clynes and Kline in their original definition of cybernetic (Clynes and Kline, 1960). I choose, however, to refer to cybernetic as Haraway's C3I (command-control-communication-intelligence), which she argues is the essential criteria for modern war (1991: 150), and I argue the C3I definitions cover the requirements needed to define an implant as cybernetic.

I will suggest that an ICD is not only smart but might be considered a cybernetic device and is therefore quite literally putting the 'cybernetic' into 'organism' and creating a cyborg. Other cyborg scholars have given the term cyborg further academic and empirical refinement (Gray, 1995a, Pollock, 2011, Oudshoorn, 2015, Oudshoorn, 2016). Scholars in Science and Technology Studies (STS) and Body Studies acknowledge the experiential basis of cyborgisation and examine how the 'cyborg' condition is created as an empirical entity (Bjorn and Markussen, 2013, Oudshoorn, 2015). Different kinds of cyborgisation created through the implantation of modern biomedical technologies, such as the implantable cardiac defibrillator (ICD), as well as cardiac pacemakers (CP), cochlear implants (CI), deep brain stimulators (DBS) and invivo biosensors (IVB) have different functions, features and therefore different consequences for the individual they are implanted within. I turn now to begin a discussion of these points with a brief outline of the modern history of the cyborg and how he (and I mean 'he') started as a hypothetical future space-man, eventually transforming into a science-fiction nightmare, to then be adopted as a feminist liberation concept from dualistic binary categorisation challenges (Haraway, 1991). In doing so, I introduce features of implantable technologies that might lead them to be considered smart and/or cybernetic, arguing that the latter eclipses all the features of the former. I compare the everyday cyborgs, to alternative versions of the cyborg (the space-man, the science-fiction monster and cyborg-as-liberator (Haddow et al., 2015)), ending with a discussion of the vulnerabilities caused by creating a techno-organic hybrid both in terms of alienation and a lack of human agency. First, however, I establish why I advocate for the use of the term 'everyday cyborg'.

Why everyday?

Adding the word 'everyday' as a prefix to the term 'cyborg' is important for a variety of reasons. First, the term 'cyborg' is hardly ever used in medical or health circles, despite both the acceptance and reliance on implantable medical technologies such as ICDs that can be considered as cybernetic. This may be due to the typical portrayal of the cyborg as monsters in film and literature, and therefore the first reason for the addition of the prefix 'everyday' signals that the 'everyday cyborg' is very different to the literature or film monster version that inhabits nightmares and I will discuss further below.

Second, there is a greater variety of implantable medical devices that have smart or cybernetic functionalities that are increasingly being relied upon on a day-by-day basis by clinicians and health professionals to save and improve the lives of individuals. The inclusion of the prefix 'everyday' is broad enough to capture the diversity of experiences from different cyborgisation processes. Reviewing research with those who have different types of smart technologies, I explore whether it can be considered 'smart' (autonomy, intelligence and responsive) as well as having features that overlap with 'cybernetic' and fulfill the C3I (Haraway, 1991).

As I will show, everyday cyborgs implanted with an ICD have additional concerns when compared to other cardiac patients relating to the vulnerabilities that are created by living life with a heart device. The ICD cybernetic system has an intimacy due to its being inside the body; an intimacy with the body that simultaneously makes it beyond the reach and control of the individual it functions within. Ironically, although the ICD might be physically out of reach of the everyday cyborg, recent policy and newspaper reports suggest that the communicative aspect of the cybernetic device makes it within reach of hackers, vulnerable to hacking by others (either through accessing data about the physiological processes or changing the device's cybernetic functions to harm the everyday cyborg).

Third and relatedly, I use the adjective 'everyday' to describe the 'new normal' or 'the new different' of living as a medically created cyborg, which, as I will show, is an achievement that cannot be taken for granted and requires acclimatisation to (Das, 2010). 'Everyday cyborgs' point to the new vulnerabilities for individuals who are created through the process of cyborgisation itself, and I will devote discussion of this moving forward. Fourth, emphasising the everyday answers the plea by medical sociologists to examine less attractive technoscience options that involve the 'subtle restructuring of identities':

> As to the medical technologies that await our investigation, we would like to repeat our plea for the seemingly mundane, 'infrastructural' technologies ... that do not have the immediate attraction of reproductive-technologies, HIV-AIDS, or genetics. It is often in the seemingly 'technical' matters that deeply relevant, social issues are 'hidden' – such as inclusion/exclusions of certain groups or voices, of the subtle restructuring of patients' or professionals' identities.
>
> (Timmermans and Berg, 2003: 108)

'Mundane' and 'hidden' is important for discussions about the creation of everyday cyborgs, not least because the implants are literally hidden inside the body, but because much of what is discussed in popular culture, academic discourse and policy circles about cyborgs (Nuffield Council on Bioethics, 2013) do not focus on what a routine day is like for some, and fewer review the 'technological mediatedness of human subjectivity' (Schraube, 2009). So, fifth, by reclaiming the cyborg for the everyday, social issues that are previously 'hidden' can be made visible.

The everyday cyborgs, I will argue, are created within social structures that create and maintain discriminatory practices; creating cyborgs therefore reifies and does not challenge existing inequalities in a cyborg society. I will outline how feminist science and technology scholar Donna Haraway described the cyborg as a 'cybernetic organism, a hybrid of machine and organism, a creature

of social reality as well as a creature of fiction' (1991: 119) to liberate individuals from the structures that constrain them; structures
that we created. Taking the lead from Haraway (1991) who uses
the cyborg as a means by which boundaries between non-human
animals and humans, the physical and the non-physical and animal-
human/machines can be dissolved, she argues for a need to focus
upon the way relations are socially structured and historically
constituted rather than solely on the technology itself (1991: 165).
Then Haraway deploys the cyborg as a positive feminist metaphor
as highlighting and simultaneously invalidating dualistic modes of
thought.

Finally, the last reason to use the term 'everyday cyborg' is that
it opens up a discussion of the gendering of the everyday cyborg
showing that the practice of cyborgisation in operating theatres
and hospitals reflects the male dominance found in science or
horror fiction about cyborgs as well as life. Hence, the value of
appropriating the term everyday cyborg encompasses the social
stratification of cyborgisation, which benefits one sub-section of
the population over another and it is, therefore, a necessary termin-
ology to identify and reveal these hidden discriminatory practices.
Cyborgisation is inevitable and is due in large part to the ever-
increasing need to repair the human body with an ever-increasing
array of technoscientific solutions in the form of implantable medical devices.

From outer space to an inside place

While speculating upon the future needs of individuals to survive
space travel, the term 'cyborg' was first introduced by researchers
Clynes and Kline, in their 1960s article 'Cyborgs and Space'. Their
implantable auto-biotechnologies included osmotic pumps to
deliver drugs, and electrical stimulation of both the heart and brain
would be required as well as standard homeostatic systems relating
to pH balance, nutrition, and glucose levels. As they stated, '[F]or
the exogenously extended organizational complex functioning as
an integrated homeostatic system unconsciously, we propose the
term "Cyborg"' (Clynes and Kline, 1960). They continue: '[T]he
Cyborg deliberately incorporates exogenous components extending

the self-regulatory control function of the organism in order to adapt it to new environments' (1960: 27). They predicted that the body of these space travellers would need a closed-loop feedback mechanism to regulate responses in space's inhospitable environment. In Clynes' original conception of the cyborg and others since then, these technological adaptations and implantations to the human body are seen as broadly acceptable, relatively risk-free and largely unproblematic for the individual. It was thought that the additions to the body required by the men during space exploration would not affect their identity. The adaptations would not necessarily affect who the men were. Indeed, as Clynes went on to suggest years later in the foreword to Halacy's *Cyborg: Evolution of the Superman*:

> Will this (cyborg) change our fundamental nature? Not much more than glasses or iron lungs change it. The difference is merely that instead of using external or *attached* prosthetic devices, the man-made devices are now to be *incorporated* into the regulatory feedback chains – the homeostatic mechanisms that keep us viable for such an astonishingly long time.
>
> (Clynes in Halacy, 1965: 8, emphasis original)

In this understanding, cybernetic alterations to the body do not affect the individual's subjectivity or relationships with others. Key to the original conception of the term cyborg is the regulation and surveillance of the body without the person necessarily being aware of it (Halacy, 1965: 75).

So according to the visions of Clynes and Kline, life on other planets could be accomplished by 'altering man's (sic) bodily functions to … artifact-organism systems which would extend man's unconscious, self-regulatory controls are one possibility' (1960: 26). However, Clynes and Kline's 'cyborg-in-space' is now arguably a present-day and everyday actuality. A trip to outer space is not needed to create the cyborg, because a cyborg is created when 'the exogenously extended organizational complex functioning as an integrated homeostatic system' takes the form of implantable medical devices that are placed inside human bodies. This, I go on to argue, creates 'everyday cyborgs' through the insertion of smart medical devices that have cybernetic capabilities, as is the case with ICDs.

Cyborgs and grinders

Implantable medical technologies can be defined as cybernetic in Clynes and Kline's (1965) original definition as a closed feedback system. For example, an ICD can sense an arrhythmia, which is an abnormally fast heart rate. It then reacts by setting off a series of small electrical shocks termed 'cardioversion', attempting to stop the rapid heart rate. The ICD then re-senses and evaluates whether a more considerable shock is required to 'defibrillate' the heart to stop the life-threatening rhythm. This is a *shock* as it is both painful and generally unexpected for the individual. The firing of an ICD imposes a 'dual shock' in many cases; there is the emotional or psychological shock of its sudden discharge and comprehension combined with the physical shock (i.e., the immediate, painful sensation) of its function. Later, the events are communicated to health professionals remotely from the device or through investigation by clinicians.

Arguably, an ICD is cybernetic because of its control over the heartbeat, its ability to enact differing commands and then communicate the subsequent events. The ICD is a closed-loop system that does not accept or require any input from the individual with whom they are implanted (whereas open-loop systems such as glucose monitors do and are more accessible to the wearer) (Ransford et al., 2014). Rather the original description of a closed feedback system appears to fulfil Norbert Wiener's classic definition of 'cybernetics', from the Greek word 'kybernutos' meaning 'governor' of a system (Wiener, 1961) and can be paraphrased in terms as 'the device's ability to function autonomously'. That is, without human intervention.

The ICD's closed feedback loop system is cybernetic in the original definition as well as fulfilling Haraway's (1991) C3I (command-control-communication-intelligence) criteria that she mentions but does not develop. Therefore, swallowing a pill or riding a bike does not make someone a cyborg, although Clynes at one point suggested that 'once you learn how to do these things automatically [ride a bike] the bike becomes almost a part of you'. He termed this as becoming almost a cyborg, but more of 'a simple cyborg' (Gray, 1995b: 49). The cyborg may be distinguishable from current-day biohackers and grinders – those whose bodies are modified by the individual. The rise of biohackers and so-called 'grinders' whose modifications range from Radio Frequency Identity Devices (RFID) and magnets implanted into fingertips bypass the biomedical expert system. In such cases, and given these implants have limited activity, permanency and bodily depths, they may be better conceptualised as being closer to tattoos rather than cybernetic systems (Radcliffe, 2011). In cases of hacking medical devices such as CIs or glucose monitors, this has occurred because the individual has been able to hack the devices' open feedback systems, accessibility that implants such as ICDs do not offer. Moreover, such practices raise questions about who owns the implants and whose responsibility it is to be able to modify them and who is to blame should they malfunction (Quigley and Ayihongbe, 2018).

Academics such as Kevin Warwick began experimenting with electrical neural implants attached to his nervous system via his arm so that he could then control a robot arm on the other side of the room (Warwick, 2003, Warwick et al., 2003, Warwick, 2004, Warwick, 2008). Some artists such as Stelarc and Orlan experiment in modifying their bodies in more permanent and visible ways. The Spanish artist Neil Harbisson who has an extreme form of colour blindness uses an antenna device he calls an 'eye-orb' that he had permanently implanted into his skull, which vibrates differentially, causing him to feel different colours.[1] These activities all share elements of human agency and choice that is not shared by those whose modifications are implantable and are medically required to improve both the quality and longevity of life.

Smart and cybernetic? Creating other 'everyday cyborgs'

In 2015 colleagues and I wrote two articles about how to define 'smart' technologies. We suggested that technology might have characteristics that were autonomous, responsive and sensitive:

> Increased smartness can be about increased automation (quicker responses which minimise role of clinician/patient), and it can be linked to the complexity of what is being sensed and responded to (e.g., measuring multiple variables which may be technologically difficult to measure), processing and delivering an appropriate response. The importance of closed loop emphasises autonomy as a

main condition of smartness (autonomy/automation) as well as complexity of responsiveness.

(Haddow, Harmon and Gilman, 2016: 217)

At that time, we had not considered whether smart could also be considered as cybernetic or what the relationship between smart and cybernetic might be. However, there are other implantable devices apart from ICDs that are either used or in development that partly fulfil features of 'smart'. Given that cybernetic systems C3I overlap with elements of smart (e.g. autonomy, intelligence or responsiveness), some implantable medical technologies such as CPs, DBSs, CIs and IVBs might be termed cybernetic as well as smart which I turn now to briefly review.

Pacemakers for the heart and brain

A cardiac pacemaker (CP) can regulate and pace the heartbeat, effectively pacing the heart from an abnormally slow rate called a 'bradycardia', with a series of small electrical charges. It is sensitive to the speed and rhythm of the heart and can discharge when it senses a slow rate but not when the heart is regularly beating. CPs collect data about the functioning of the immediate environment (e.g., the heart) and provide therapy (e.g., releasing electrical pulses and/or an electric shock) in response and so are viewed as more 'active' than, say, heart valve replacements. CPs share many of the features of an ICD (and indeed many ICDs have pacing features) and are therefore an example of smart technology featuring autonomy, intelligence and responsive ability. With the addition of functions that might include wireless communications such as those an ICD has, they may also be termed cybernetic. Interestingly, when the first studies were done with those individuals who had CP implanted, issues arose regarding body integrity and image as with individuals implanted with ICDs years later (of which more discussion below) (Green and Moss, 1969).

Frequently presented as a 'pacemaker for the brain', deep brain stimulators (DBSs) comprise electrodes implanted in the brain, a pulse generator implanted in the chest (near the collarbone), and a subcutaneous wire connecting them. Intended to alleviate tremors, stiffness and slowness caused by Parkinson's disease, reports suggest that DBS may have implications for improving lung function, memory and mood disorders such as depression. DBSs have been the subject of intense investigation as studies have uncovered: 1) very different expectations for, and tolerances about, chronic illnesses and the side-effects of their treatment, 2) the variety and progression of emotional response to DBS and 3) the need for greater cooperation between stakeholders to create realistic public perceptions of DBS. DBSs can significantly improve symptoms and like CP and ICDs take control out of the hands of the everyday cyborg. Because they are fully implantable and cannot be reached by the individual, they create new challenges and vulnerabilities (Gardner, 2013, Klaming and Haselager, 2013, Gardner et al., 2017, Gardner and Warren, 2019). DBSs have also been the subject of legal concern, for they have been known to cause significant personality change, which can have implications for capacity (Klaming and Haselager, 2013). Others suggest that they do not necessarily alter subjectivity despite the modern era's emphasis on the brain as the location of self noted throughout this book. This appears to confirm the 'ambiguity of embodiment' discussed elsewhere that personal identity is more embodied, relational and dynamic and that individuals are not reducible to their brains, despite the necessity of having one (Lipsman and Glannon, 2012, Gardner, 2013, Kraemer, 2013, Gilbert, 2017, Gardner and Warren, 2019, Gardner et al., 2019).

In terms of smart functionality, cochlear implants (CIs) can provide a sense of sound to those who are profoundly deaf or extremely hard-of-hearing. CIs do not restore 'normal hearing', but instead replace it by interacting with the environment and the auditory nerve. They are penetrative but not truly implantable as are CPs or DBS. An external part comprising a microphone, a speech processor and a transmitter sits behind the ear, and an internal component comprising an electrode array is surgically placed within the ear to stimulate the auditory nerve. The person can remove the outside monitor from their ear; they have an element of control over CI – a human operator can still control the device. Although not due to a lack of human control, CI recipients report that the device can cause them stress and vulnerability (Chorost, 2005). Partly, this is due to expectations about the device being unmet; the difficulty in tuning the devices; and continuing communication problems associated with childhood deafness (Stinson and Buckley, 2013).

The device can also lead to 'non-auditory stimulation' – where nerves around the site are stimulated by the electrical energy, and this can lead to facial twitching (Gray et al., 1998). Moreover, as Blume argues (1999), little consultation with the Deaf community meant that the development of the technology was initially met with varying degrees of resistance, rejection and ambivalence depending on individual circumstances (Stinson and Buckley, 2013).

Finally, in-vivo biosensors (IVBs) are an example of an implantable medical technology that is currently in development to enhance the accuracy of radiotherapy treatment for cancerous tumours (Haddow et al., 2015). Many tumours can be treated effectively with radiotherapy; however, some are stubbornly radio resistant. Biosensors may be able to demonstrate resistance by undertaking biological measurements of the tumour environment, assessing whether real-time fluctuations in oxygen and pH levels could be exploited to optimise the timing of treatment to overcome radiotherapy resistance. Our early social science research with recovering prostate cancer patients demonstrates a willingness to accept in vivo biosensors and enthusiasm for a more ambitious functionality that goes beyond the current ambition of a beacon system (i.e., identifying the timing and location for radiotherapy and providing information about the environment) leaning more towards an IVB that is a long-term surveillance system alerting when there is a reappearance of cancer tumours (Haddow et al., 2015). However, there was an undercurrent of ambivalence reported and periods of 'acclimatisation' or of becoming accustomed were mentioned. Indeed, initial willingness to have an IVB varied depending on the circumstances around their implantation and the concomitant evaluation of what will be lost and gained by the men. For some, the attraction of the IVBs related to the masculine image often found in *fictionalised* presentations of a cyborg rather than what the respondents termed a 'leaker and a bleeder'. It is these fictionalised accounts I turn to next.

Cyborg as sci-fi monster

Modern-day implantable medical devices exhibit a range of smart and cybernetic functionality, and there appears to be a willingness of some to become an 'everyday cyborg' under certain circumstances.

However, using the term as a way to describe people is controversial due in large part to the cyborg's depiction in the genres of science and horror fiction. This is because as Turkle (2011) notes: '[W]e approach our technologies through a battery of advertising and media narratives; it is hard to think above the din'. In the public imagination the cyborg is a science-fiction monster born in the image of a technologically enhanced organism as portrayed in a multitude of books and films (Oetler, 1995).

Often the distinction between cyborgs, androids and robots is conflated; even by Clynes when he expressed horror at what his 'cyborg-in-space' had become in the science-fiction genre: 'Well at first I was amused and then I was horrified because it was a total distortion ... This recent film with this Terminator, with Schwarzenegger playing this thing – dehumanized the concept completely' (Gray, 1995b: 47). Perhaps Clynes might not have worried so much if he knew that 'Terminator' was not, strictly speaking, a cyborg according to his and Kline's criteria. Robots are fully mechanical, artificial, sophisticated devices with no organic elements, whereas an android, such as 'Terminator', is a robot that bears an external resemblance to a human or non-human living organism; neither is necessarily the cyborg that Clynes refers to.

Setting aside these differences when comparing fiction and reality, one of the most obvious distinctions between the science-fiction monster and the original Clynes cyborg version is that in the case of the former the cybernetic technology negatively affects the individual's subjectivity. These cyborg monsters are visible techno-organic hybrids typically, but not always, shown as being incapable of *feeling* or demonstrating emotions – they are portrayed as being both inhuman and inhumane. In science fiction, the cyborgs are the terrifying 'Borg' in Star Trek, the 'Cybermen' in Dr Who, or Alex Murphy in 'Robocop' who are typically presented as a cyborg monster bereft of emotions and feelings.[2] These cyborg monsters generally have the physical attributes of strength and power and overt musculature co-existent with the dominant Western idea of masculinity (Connell, 1995). Gray argues that gendering of the cyborg is not just prevalent in science fiction or even in the 'cyborg-in-space' versions, but explicitly with the technological focus and dominance found, for example, in the phrase 'toys for the boys' and adaptations and control of the male penis for sexual attraction and intercourse (Gray, 2000). The sci-fi cyborg's technological adaptations simultaneously remove the ability for the cyborg to act humanely by adding technology to human materiality. That is, by removing human organic material and replacing or adding mechanical parts, the new techno-organic hybrid gains strength and power but at the cost of attributes such as empathy and compassion associated with being human.

The masculinity, as well as inhumanity of the fiction cyborg, is a trend that can be traced historically to the 'creature' created by a scientist 'Frankenstein' in the gothic novel by the author Mary Shelley (Shelley, [1831] 1993). A precursor to a body that is created entirely by assembling different organs, the monster created by Mary Shelley's 'Frankenstein' was a montage of materials from other human corporeal beings, but referred to as male nonetheless. In the introduction to the 1993 reprint, Jansson suggests:

> For Mary Shelley, however, two of the most important aspects of science centre upon the essential 'masculinity' of scientific thought … This 'masculinity' is most evident in the removal of any feminine element from the Creature's 'birth'; the scientific process activated by Victor excluded any sense of the humanity of the Creature.
>
> (1993: x)

Frankenstein's monster, although not a cyborg, was a visible manifestation of a monster and, similar to modern-day depictions of robots, androids and cyborgs, they also need to be visible. Baudrillard notes the societal angst created by 'invisible robots', highlighting the perceived danger to human sensibilities of not making their 'inhumanness' (or otherness) apparent:

> the substitution in question *has* to be visible: if it is to exert its fascination without creating insecurity, the robot must unequivocally reveal its nature as a mechanical prosthesis (its body is metallic, its gestures are discrete, jerky and unhuman).
>
> (Baudrillard, 1996: 129)

A cyborg is more likely to represent this 'invisible danger' being referred to insofar as the inhumanness, and the subsequent threat, is not apparent due to the cybernetics being implanted and therefore the techno-organic hybridity not being visible. The ability to perceive inhumanness appears important so that the artificial exterior and the difference between 'us' and 'them' is realised.

In being unable to distinguish the cyborg amongst us it arguably creates ontological insecurity and fear.

On the occasions when a female cyborg (or indeed android) is portrayed, it is generally of an overtly sexualised female entity. Her technological modifications focus on specific aspects of the female biology such as the bikini area and on feminine traits such as the ability to listen or to be more emotionally literate. In the film *Ex Machina* released in 2015 and directed by Alex Garland, 'Ava' an android, passes the Turing test by using her emotional intelligence, femininity and (pseudo) submissiveness. Ava is from a long line of female androids, from 'Maria' in Fritz Lang's *Metropolis* to the film *Blade Runner*, featuring 'Pris' (the sex pleasure model) and Rachel (who exhibits human emotions) to '7 of 9' in *Star Trek Voyager*. In 2015, the UK Channel 4 series *Humans* featured the 'synths' with the mostly young, female characters as androids presented as either sex-bots or care-bots looking after the family.

A cyborg's mother – the liberator

The gendering of the android and the cyborg says as much about gender dynamics in present-day society (e.g. the strong rational male versus the emotional, sexual caring female) as it does about the future status of robots, androids and cyborgs.[3] The gendering of the cyborg is dealt with critically in STS literature (Haraway, 1991, Gray, 1995a, Hayles, 1995) and feminist STS literature (Penley, Ross and Haraway, 1990, Kirkup et al., 1999, Henwood, Kennedy and Miller, 2001). In this literature, another version of the cyborg emerges which is most well-known by the feminist philosopher and social theorist Haraway, in her important paper 'The Cyborg Manifesto' (1991). According to Haraway, the cyborg is a 'cybernetic organism, a hybrid of machine and organism, a creature of social reality as well as a creature of fiction' (1991: 119).

Haraway's cyborg is a means in which boundaries between animals and humans, the physical and the non-physical and animal-human/machines, are dissolved (Haraway, 2003). As she argues, this is not about focusing purely on the technology per se but upon the socially structured relations amongst people that have been historically constituted (1991: 165). Simply put, this is the way things are because this is the way they have been. The cyborg, for Haraway, I believe, is an ironic representation and abstraction to show how we are constructors of our cages – and the existence of the cyborg indicates the possibility of this to be different. She is using the cyborg as a tool in her 'ironic' Manifesto. Perhaps her Manifesto is, at first sight, a more playful one than a Marxist one, but its message nonetheless is a serious one. Haraway's cyborg is an abstract representation that is needed to challenge existing schema regarding how in terms of cyborgisation the existence of gender division now requires subverting.

Haraway deploys the cyborg as a positive feminist metaphor and as a means of highlighting and invalidating the inherent impurity of any dualistic system thought or mode. The cyborg is ahistorical and post-gender with an ability to liberate from classificatory categories. Haraway used the term as an ontological challenge to the gender dualisms that carried inherent within them the power that causes an imbalance that is generally subverting the 'woman'. The cyborg is a challenge to modern society but one that we are responsible for:

> A cyborg body is not innocent; it was not born in a garden; it does not seek unitary identity and so generate antagonistic dualisms without end (or until the world ends); it takes irony for granted ... Intense pleasure in skill, machine skill, ceases to be a sin, but an aspect of embodiment ... We can be responsible for machines; they do not dominate or threaten us. We are responsible for boundaries; we are they.
>
> (1991: 180)

However, machines are dominating and threatening, and technology is a reflection and is not (yet) a challenge to discriminatory practices. At the time Haraway published her *Cyborg Manifesto* in 1985, many people were already living with technologically augmented bodies for medical therapy. The unevenness of an 'invasion', charting who will be affected, and with what and why, is neither well-documented or understood. The everyday cyborg is not yet an icon of liberation envisioned by Haraway (1991, 2003). The everyday cyborg may reflect current socio-technological developments and biomedical practices that are reifying existing inequalities in a cyborg society. This takes a concrete form when analysing data about who becomes an everyday cyborg as I turn to next.

Mending broken hearts

In the UK, government figures from the Office for National Statistics show that ischaemic heart disease is the leading cause of death in men, and the second leading cause of death in women of all ages (2001 to 2018) (Office of National Statistics, 2018). A heart attack causes most deaths from heart disease. Heart disease causes a plaque or a wax to build up in the arteries of the heart whose primary responsibility is to supply oxygen to the heart muscles that cause the heart to beat. Reducing the blood flow means clots are more likely, leading to angina and heart attacks. Those individuals who survive a heart attack may sustain some further form of long-term damage to their heart. Damage from a heart attack results in damage to the heart muscle, and this can eventually result in heart failure. A previous heart attack may scar heart structures, preventing it from working correctly (so-called 'myocardial infarction').

Moreover, having suffered a prior heart attack can be linked to the occurrence of a sudden cardiac arrest (SCA). The difference between a heart attack and an SCA is demonstrated best by using the image of a house whereby a heart attack is akin to a 'blockage in the pipes problem', and an SCA is an electrical fault. However, the former can also lead to the latter.

An SCA, therefore, is not the same as a heart attack, although it can be caused by having had one. An SCA is produced by cells in the ventricles of the heart (the left bottom chamber of the heart) firing electrical signals that cause the heart to beat faster than usual. This is known as ventricular tachycardia. In tachycardia, the heart beats at 120–200 beats a minute. Electrical impulses start firing haphazardly from different sites in the heart. The tachycardia can worsen into ventricular fibrillation when the heart beats in an abnormal rhythm that cannot be sustained by the body; the heart 'fibrillates' or quivers instead of beating and pumping blood. Ashcroft, quoting the 16th-century anatomist Vesalius, draws parallels between a fibrillating heart and a 'writhing bag of worms' (Ashcroft, 2012). If this is not remedied by a strong electrical shock to defibrillate the heart, then a cardiac arrest will follow. The UK's National Institute of Clinical Excellence (NICE, 2014) suggests that of the 70,000 sudden cardiac deaths in England and Wales in 2010, almost 80 per cent were caused by heart arrhythmias (NICE, 2014: 5).

Heart conditions can be treated or prevented by a range of medications but also by the use of implantable cardiac devices. The ICD is viewed as the gold standard treatment for the avoidance of death from cardiac arrhythmias. Most cardiac mechanical therapies are devices used as a permanent intervention and are viewed as a successful, even underused, therapy (Burns et al., 2005). Once implanted, these devices are rarely removed, which can raise ethical issues around if and when communication of end-of-life decisions should be made (Kelley, Mehta and Reid, 2008) as I shall discuss later.

ICDs are increasingly sophisticated, and with the introduction of cardiac resynchronisation devices (CRTs) there is an additional ability to pace both ventricles of the heart in individuals who have advanced heart failure (CRT-P) and have the ability to discharge shocks (CRT-D). An ICD is relatively inactive and is in a low power mode to conserve battery, but it does have an ability to emit small electric shocks to convert a rapid heart rhythm similar to a CP. ICDs, unlike CPs discussed earlier, can treat many different types of arrhythmias that are fast (tachycardia) and slow (bradycardia) and can discharge larger electrical shocks when pacing and cardioversion has not stopped the arrhythmia. The ICD can discharge shocks up to 40 joules, which is much lower than an external defibrillator in a hospital could give (100–360j).[4] Most people who suffer an SCA are unlikely to survive unless CPR (chest compression and rescue breathing) is given immediately or an electric shock is administered. Estimates are that only 7 per cent of adults who experience a ventricular arrhythmia out of hospital are expected to survive (NICE, 2014: 5).

Individuals who have experienced an arrhythmia will be implanted with an ICD. This is to protect them from a recurrence and is termed 'secondary prevention'. An ICD can be implanted electively for prophylactic reasons when a patient is at high risk of a future arrhythmia but has not yet suffered one. NICE guidelines suggest that people who have conditions such as Brugada syndrome, arrhythmogenic right ventricular dysplasia, hypertrophic cardiomyopathy or QT syndrome are recommended to have an ICD prophylactically (NICE, 2014). These people may not have experienced a cardiac arrest but are deemed as being at a high risk of lethal arrhythmias due to the existing clinical pathology and hence are fitted for reasons of primary prevention.

Made by men for men

The UK's audit system of ICDs and CP uses data to explore how different areas in the UK are performing in terms of the number of active cardiac device procedures being undertaken compared to the national averages (Buxton et al., 2006). In the UK, a Health Technology Assessment conducted in 2006 highlighted that approximately 80 per cent of ICDs were implanted into men and 20 per cent into women (Buxton et al., 2006). More recent and additional data on age and ethnicity is not yet available in a consistent form in the UK. In the US, such data is collected in a National ICD Registry. A published report based on an analysis of this data from 2006 to 2009 demonstrates that ICDs were more commonly implanted into white men who had not yet suffered a cardiac arrest so the procedure was undergone for primary prophylactic reasons:

Table 3.1 National ICD Registry (2006–2009): demographics, ICD indication

Age, mean (yrs)	68.1 ± 12.8
Male/female (%)	73.8/26.2
Race (%)	
White	82.8
Black/African American	12.1
Asian	1.0
American Indian/Alaska Native	0.4

Native Hawaiian	0.1
Other	3.4
Hispanic	4.9
Total implants (N)	486,025
ICD indication (N, %)	
Primary prevention	378,363 (77.9)
Secondary prevention	107,662 (22.2)
Primary insurance payor (%)	
Medicare/Medicaid	67.7
Other payor	32.3

Source: Hammill et al., 2010

Of the procedures conducted in the United States, 77.9 per cent were implanted into white men to prevent them having an SCA compared to only 22.2 per cent implanted into women. Undoubtedly, some of the differences in ICD implantation rates between men and women are caused by 1) a lower incidence of heart disease in women and 2) women presenting with symptoms of heart disease at a later age. Contextualised within the general ageing of the population (and of women in particular), more women than men die of cardiovascular disease in the US (Wenger, 2004: 558). Heart disease is the primary cause of death for both men and women in the US and disproportionately women of colour.[5] Further, women are less likely to be treated for heart disease, and this is partly due to the fact that they are less likely to present with symptoms such as STEMI (ST-Elevation Myocardial Infarction) which account for approximately 25–40 per cent of myocardial infarctions in the US (O'Gara et al., 2013). A review of research by Yarnoz and Curtis (2006) argues that 'the male dominance in device therapy can be rationalized from the higher proportion of men with CAD and serious systolic heart failure' as:

> Women have a lower incidence of CAD [coronary artery disease] and tend to present with this disease at a later age than men. Advancing age might *make implantation in females a less attractive therapeutic option compared with younger male counterparts.*
>
> (2006: 297, my emphasis)[6]

Women tend to suffer from sudden cardiac death and myocardial infarctions roughly 20 years later in the life course than men do so the case for ICD implantation is evaluated on who is more likely to benefit, and the answer is that it is not an older woman but a younger man.

This social stratification of ICD implantations suggests that there is a form of 'cyborg sexism' when women who may benefit from ICD implantation are not offered one. Partly this discrimination may be due to technologising only the 'bikini area' of women, for example, with breast implants and contraceptive devices and, in the more recently publicised case of vaginal meshes, partly because what is assumed for men is (wrongly) applied to women (Wise, 2016, Wise, 2017, Rimmer, 2018). Some early evidence suggests a gender disparity concerning the implantation of DBS, and researchers argue it may be due to women's preference not to be implanted (Shpiner et al., 2019). However, women fitted with contraceptive implants demonstrate a willingness to be implanted despite other alternative means of contraception that do not involve this procedure (Davie et al., 1996). The social stratification of cyborgisation or 'cyborg sexism' may remain an on-going concern.

An ambiguity of benefiting from cyborgisation – a new vulnerability?

The effects that ICDs have on individuals and their significant others is also troubling. Most psychological studies[7] conducted with ICD patients repeatedly document the prevalence of anxiety, depression and even anger in the ICD population. However, this data cannot explain whether these emotions are a result of the implantation of the ICD, the activation of an ICD, discharging a shock or were pre-existing tendencies relating to the nature of the heart condition (Green and Moss, 1969, Tchou et al., 1989, Sakensa, 1994, Duru et al., 2001, Bunch et al., 2004, Kuhl et al., 2006, Birnie et al., 2007, Bunch et al., 2008, Pedersen et al., 2008, Yuhas et al., 2012, Vriesendorp et al., 2013, Asad et al., 2014).

Studies of men's experiences with coronary heart disease show similar issues like those reported by ICD patients, for example, from a 'loss of physical strength, emotional health, paid work, financial security, independence, self-esteem, control, leisure activities, social life, pleasures (alcohol, a particular food, smoking, sex) and social life' (Emslie and Hunt, 2009: 177). All cardiac patients may develop some illness identity dislocations as they suffer from having heart disease, condition or arrest as well as from a near-death experience (Charmaz, 1995). An obvious starting point, however, is to compare features specific to everyday cyborgs that differentiate them from other heart condition patients. That is, the implantation of a cybernetic device into their body and its possible activation.

Implantation: outside-in

The surgery for the ICD (and CP) is generally conducted under local anaesthetic with a sedative given to the patient. The ICD's generator or battery is in a sealed case and inserted into the left-hand side of the pectoral chest with the leads fed down by the surgeon into the heart's atrium and ventricle. The leads or electrodes are vital to allowing the monitoring of heart rate and rhythms and delivering the shocks. This electrical circuitry monitors heart rhythm; makes the decision whether or not to administer a shock; delivers the shock; then monitors the response, judging whether more therapy is required and hence why, as I argued earlier, it can be considered cybernetic.[8] ICDs can usually distinguish between arrhythmias in differing chambers of the heart, such as atrial fibrillation and ventricular tachycardia. This is important because atrial fibrillation causes a rapid heart rate but rarely requires a shock. The level of arrhythmia that the ICD detects is set by an electrophysiologist during implantation and can be modified (Vriesendorp et al., 2013).

The ICD is in a liminal location both in and on the body. It is placed inside the body and yet can be perceived on the skin as the generator causes a bump or a silhouette on the skin where it is implanted (Dalibert, 2016). It can both be touched and felt on the inside (integrity) and outside (image) of the body. An ICD and a CP can compromise the body's *integrity*, a term I introduced earlier referring to the inside of the body as a component of the 'Triad of I'. Some of Dickerson's participants told her, 'it's a foreign object in my body, close to my heart' and 'I need to get used to its presence' and 'I am being controlled and regulated by a machine (Dickerson, 2002: 365). One participant discussed how she had delayed implantation: '[I] fought it for a long time. The thought of having some kind of mechanical thing in my body turned me off and I didn't want it. I resisted it [pause] just because it's something mechanical and not natural' (Beery et al., 2002: 16). Beery and colleagues describe how eventually all acknowledged the cardiac device as 'part of me', but it had not been without challenges (Beery et al., 2002). Nicknames were often used to refer to the device ranging from 'best friend' to 'foreign object', 'gift' and 'little sucker', which the authors argue are indicative that the women gradually acclimatised to the pacemaker.

Some studies have shown that women are more likely to report higher levels of body image concerns than men (Starrenburg et al., 2014) perhaps by causing particularly practical problems for women: 'I can't wear underwired bras anymore' (Tagney, 2003: 199). Other studies show that body image affects men and women equally, as the ICD's silhouette serves as a reminder of the purpose of the ICD, whose function is to save lives and is, therefore, evidence of the everyday cyborg's mortality:

> Every time I look in the mirror I think, oh, you've got an ICD in your chest. There's a physical manifestation of what happened to me. It's something that happened inside my body, but I can see it every day when I take a shower. I look in the mirror and I see a little lump. Yeah, I think about what happened to me every day.
>
> (Pollock, 2011: 100)

For Beery's cardiac pacemaker and Dickerson's ICD participants, an initial feeling of loss of control eventually transformed into a conditional acceptance (Dickerson, 2002).

Shocking functionality

ICDs provide painful shocks at unpredictable times – the defibrillation mentioned above. In many cases, these are 'dual shocks' as there is the physical shock (i.e., the sudden and painful sensation) of its function but also an unexpected shock. These shocks are likened to being 'kicked in the chest by horse' and scoring a 6 in a pain-scale of 0–10 (Pelletier et al., 2002, Ahmad et al., 2000). The ICD shocks represent a near-death experience for the individual in terms of the fatal consequences if it had not fired, but one where the odds were against them in terms of their chances of survival without it. A review of research in 1999 suggested:

> ICD-specific fears and symptoms of anxiety (e.g. excessive, worry, physiological arousal) are the most common psychological symptoms experienced by ICD recipients, with approximately 13–38% of recipients experiencing diagnosable levels of anxiety. Depressive symptoms are reported at rates that are generally consistent with other cardiac populations. Although the incidence of psychological disorders appears to be similar to that found in general cardiac populations, specific ICD-related concerns such as fear of shock, fear of device malfunction, fear of death and fear of embarrassment have been identified.
>
> (Sears et al., 1999: 481)

A recent systematic review of the literature reiterates the findings that ICD patients are at an increased risk of mental health problems relating to depression, anxiety and panic attacks. Research with ICD patients leads Oudshoorn to suggest that, 'Having a machine inside your body without knowing when or where it may jolt you induces feelings of disbelief and anxiety' (Oudshoorn, 2016: 8). The more shocks experienced by the individual, the higher the level of anxiety (White, 2002, Withell, 2006). Of women who receive ICDs, it is reported they suffer more from increased anxiety and concerns about the ICD relative to men regardless of whether they had experienced shocks (Spindler et al., 2009). Some researchers suggest that moods, including depression and anger, cause arrhythmic events (Dunbar et al., 1999, Lampert et al., 2002). Although Whang et al. (2005) suggest that depression is an indicator for appropriate shocks, while others suggest that there is a risk of ventricular arrhythmia after implantable defibrillator treatment in anxious Type D patients (van den Broek et al., 2009). Oudshoorn suggests that cyborgisation created by the implantation of an ICD leads to two new types of vulnerability 'as an internal rather than an external threat and as harm you may try to anticipate but can never escape' (Oudshoorn, 2016: 267). Vulnerability is caused by the embeddedness of the technology, creating a paradox of both closeness and distance along with an inability to control the device's functionality. As will be shown in the next chapter, however, the everyday cyborg believes they can create the circumstances in which the ICD has shocked them.

Identity and relationships

Issues around lack of control as well as body image and integrity appear to be important issues of the everyday cyborg. However, effects can go beyond the individual's body to alter the relationships they have with others, as well as the relations others have with them. 'Over-protectiveness' of significant others is often complained about in research with ICD patients (Dougherty, 1997, Eckert and Jones, 2002, Dougherty, Pyper and Benoliel, 2004, Insurers, 2004, Palacios-Cena et al., 2011). Dickerson's informants suggested, 'It has taken time for those around me to realize I can handle "stressful" scenarios ... They are always worried that my "heart" is not OK ... I think it's critical to educate others' (Dickerson, 2002: 367). This is a common complaint in those who have suffered coronary heart disease, so over-protectiveness may not be unique to having an ICD fitted (Emslie and Hunt, 2009: 177). Indeed, there is mention of a reduction in physical exertions including sexual (Craney et al., 1997) with reports of only 40 per cent of individuals resuming sexual relations (Steinke et al., 2005). Figures reported in the 'Sexual Activity and Cardiovascular Disease: A Scientific Statement From the American Heart Association' report that the risk of cardiac arrest during sexual activity is small (0.6–1.7 per cent) (Levine et al., 2012). It is noted:

> partner overprotectiveness and the fear of shock with sexual activity are important concerns for the patient and his or her partner. Accordingly, sexual activity often decreases after ICD implantation. The sexual partner is not believed to be at risk from defibrillation if the ICD discharges during sexual activity.
>
> (Levine, 2012: 6)

So cyborgisation caused by implanting ICDs in individuals is a matter of concern for the individual and equally important is the effects that go beyond their identity to alter relationships with others. There is, however, a risk that others may seek to affect the ICD with malicious intent as I turn to next.

Hacking

In 2007, the United States vice-president Dick Cheney had the wireless function of his pacemaker disabled by his cardiologist who is reported as suggesting: 'It seemed to me to be a bad idea for the vice-president to have a device that maybe somebody on a rope line or in the next hotel room or downstairs might be able to get into – hack into.'[9]

Cardiac devices such as CPs and ICDs, are getting smaller, smarter and more interconnected, and accompanying this arises concerns about data security and system hacking. Unlike insulin pumps which are an open-loop system and can accept patient input (and indeed as shown previously are hackable by the patient), ICDs are cybernetic features which are closed-loop systems. They have software to be able to sense physiological changes in the heart, to 'know' when the appropriate time to emit a shock is, as well as being able to transmit this data remotely – they are cybernetic due to the prescence of C3I. Quigley and Ayihongbe suggest that it is due to the integration of hardware and software that controls the how, when and why therapy is delivered that is integral to the everyday cyborg (Quigley and Ayihongbe, 2018). In the UK, everyday ICD cyborgs can be offered a home monitor that uploads information from their pacemaker or ICD to the hospital through the landline or wi-fi internet connections. Instead of attending a clinic for a check-up, a virtual appointment is sent that tells the everyday cyborg when to pick up the device and place it on their chest over the ICD. Information is downloaded from the ICD inside the body through the device and sent to the hospital. A programmer can interrogate the ICD from in the hospital clinic. Medtronic is one of the largest suppliers of remote ICD monitors and as it states on its website:

> The Medtronic CareLink® Network is the nation's leading remote monitoring service, connecting cardiac device patients to their clinic from home or away.* As a clinician, you have 24/7 access – via a secure Internet website – to a wide range of trended reports offering information comparable to an in-office visit.[†] These diagnostic reports can be exported to your hospital network or EHR for greater accessibility to the data and clinical documentation. In addition, you can receive Medtronic CareAlert.® Notifications which provide alerts to potential issues before they become problems.[10]

Information can include whether the device has fired or not and the amount of battery it has left (which varies depending on how many shocks it has discharged). This has led others to conclude: 'when a cardiac implant gains a wireless interface for clinical monitoring, it may expose the patient to malicious eavesdropping (a violation of privacy) or tampering' (Halperin et al., 2008b).

There are two ways that hacking can affect cardiac devices through interfering with the radio frequency enabled aspect – either through theft of data or interfering with the functionality of the device. It is alleged that an attack could be made through using EMI waveform (electromagnetic interference).

> With a carefully crafted EMI (electromagnetic interference) wave-form and an implantable defibrillator with its leads in free air, the researchers confused the ICD's sensors and tricked the ICD into delivering a defibrillation shock. (Ransford et al., 2014: 166)

As stated, 'leads in free air' appears to indicate that the ICD was not 'confused' when it was in the body. So, the attack was not made through the skin or muscle to the ICD when implanted. A report carried out for the European Commission in 2006 'Safeguards in a World of Ambient Intelligence' (SWAMI) outlines scenarios where 'remote homicide' may be possible by hacking into devices and disrupting their software or signals to give wrong treatments or prevent emergency signals being responded to (Friedewald, Lindner and Wright, 2006). Other risks include forced battery depletion (Halperin et al., 2008b) and the 'tracking of unwitting patients' (Roberts, 2011, Ransford et al., 2014: 158). This latter example relates to the specific technology of insulin pumps that are neither embedded in the body nor have a closed-looped system. Although evidence is gathering that an attack on an ICD is possible, an actual hack into an everyday cyborg's ICD to collect data or cause the device to malfunction is yet, I believe, to be unequivocally shown. Arguably, one of the largest challenges to any hacker is reaching the device that is partially submerged in the body. This is not to say that it cannot happen. There is far more evidence, however, to suggest that malfunctioning or inaccuracy of the ICD occur without necessarily being hacked.

Faults in the machine

Estimates suggest that approximately 60 per cent of ICD patients will receive a shock within their first two years (Buxton et al., 1999). Oudshoorn's (2016) review of ICD patients' accounts on social media highlights that some could anticipate or know when a shock was inappropriate or not. Inappropriate shocks occur mainly from: faults in the leads; the ICD over-sensing activity in the atrium of the heart instead of the ventricles; or the upper threshold being set too low for the individual. The ICD is more accurately described as a system, as it consists of leads and a generator. The leads that are implanted into the heart are arguably as important as the generator and battery itself; loose or broken leads can lead to inappropriate shocks or failure to cardiovert or defibrillate (Piot et al., 2015). In 2005, Medtronic undertook a voluntary recall of all 'sprint fidelis' leads because of concerns about this.

An investigation discovered that when compared to a previous version of the lead, predictions were that the sprint fidelis mortality rates would be significantly higher (Ellenbogen, Wood and Swerdlow, 2008). The issue relates to using a lead that is thin enough to make implantation easier for the surgeon (discussed in detail next in Chapter 4), but sturdy enough to be able to withstand the continued pressure from the heart's beat. In the US, others have noted that since 1990, 41 per cent of ICD and CP recalls were due to firmware malfunctions (Maisel et al., 2001). In 2018, a report of medical device recalls showed a 126 per cent increase occurring in the US, with ICD's featuring frequently on the list.[11]

There is some evidence to suggest records of ICD activity can be inaccurate or contradict the experience of shock discharge by the everyday cyborg. Research has discussed the phenomenon of nocturnal shocks as 'phantom shocks' whereby the everyday cyborg reports frequent defibrillation during sleep, but upon interrogation, the device shows no activity (House et al., 2018). As shown in Table 3.2 below, ICDs can inaccurately record the date of arrhythmia incidents occurring in 2005 rather than 2007 (Halperin et al., 2008a: 33).

Table 3.2 Arrhythmia logbook report

Episode	Date/Time	Type	Zone/Rate bpm		Therapy/ Duration
1.230	23 June 2005 19:10	Spont	VF	222	Diverted
1.229	20 June 2005 12:08	Spont	VF	216	Diverted
1.228	21 May 2007 21:22	ATR		130	??:??
1.227	21 May 2007 15:01	ATR		121	06:20 h:m
1.226	21 May 2007 15:01	ATR		119	00:45 m:s
1.225	21 May 2007 15:00	ATR		120	00:11 m:s
1.224	21 May 2007 15:00	ATR		119	00:16 m:s
1.223	21 May 2007 15:00	ATR		118	00:07 m:s
1.222	21 May 2007 14:59	ATR		119	00:09 m:s

Conclusion: the call for everyday cyborgs

The increasing acceptance and reliance on technological fixes, such as implantable cardiac defibrillators (ICDs), are a feature of today's medical systems and therapeutic regimes (Clarke et al., 2010), the consequences of which I return to later in the book. Individuals are amongst us that are having to live life with bodies modified through implanted cybernetic medical technologies. The people who are living life with their cybernetic heart devices in their hybrid bodies I call everyday cyborg. In sum, so far, I have advocated for using the term 'cyborg' while being well aware of the controversy that surrounds the term. Apart from a few notable exceptions in academic research, 'cyborg' is a term that appears to be mostly avoided. Indeed, in the past, the term may have largely been referred to without the benefit of empirical data or an argument about the need for the term. Indeed, when the term cyborg has been used variously, the most well known is the cyborg models of science-fiction monsters, which are often confused with androids. The cyborg monsters, in particular, make most people feel unable or uncomfortable to consider any other forms of cybernetic organisms. It is the case, however, that everyday cyborgs do exist whereas sci-fi monsters do not. The cultural baggage associated with the term 'cyborg' is hiding how cybernetic technology is socially stratified within the population, more available to some and not others, and thus why some groups are more likely (or not) to become an everyday cyborg. Despite Haraway's challenge and call for the cyborg to deconstruct dualisms, such as those that involve gender, the cyborg is a highly gendered trope both in science and horror fiction and, as argued here, an empirical reality.

The reference point for living as an everyday cyborg is a hybrid of a mostly fictional character and of the science-fiction caricature of a monster, not that of the original space-man [sic]. A common feature of all versions of the cyborg, however, is masculinity – male everyday cyborg, the space-man and the male cyborg sci-fi monster who transforms into an entity less human and there-fore less humane. Here similarities in the different versions of a cyborg, diverge; the everyday cyborg becomes more vulnerable, more humane and requires strategies and support to cope with the vulnerabilities. The vulnerability that everyday cyborgs are susceptible to is different from other patients who do not live life as an organic-techno hybrid, although more research is needed to see whether an everyday cyborg created by the implantation of an ICD experiences the same or different vulnerabilities as one created by a DBS, for example. An ICD is cybernetic as its cap-abilities go well beyond that of other semi-implantable technolo-gies such as CIs, and prosthetic technologies that do not have the ability to autonomously react to changes in their environment (Harmon, Haddow and Gilman, 2015, Haddow, Harmon and Gilman, 2016). Increasing the number of everyday cyborgs in society carries new challenges for a cyborg society.

Alienation on implantation

As I discussed in this chapter, creating different types of everyday cyborgs – machines in the human/cybernetics in the organism – pose different types of risks to the individual not solely on possible malfunctioning, but on the correct functioning of the technology, the bodily location of where it was implanted in, the reasons for it being implanted, the type of technology, and patient expectations of the benefits. Questions about how different types and kinds of implantable technologies or materialities affect us appear remote and distant in ordinary life and daily routines. We are embodied, and the relationship between body image, integrity and identity (my so-called 'Triad of I') is a taken-for-granted experience and rarely a source for reflection. Our bodies, to a certain extent, are 'absent' (Leder 1990). Modifying the body through implantation and transplantation, however, can draw attention to the nature of the relationship that a person has with their body; indeed, centuries ago the philosopher Descartes showed in his reflections just how divisible the person and their body is. In the Cartesian biomedical understanding of the body-person, both aspects are separate, yet it is not always clear in our everyday experience of embodiment that we are not our bodies; in fact, being a body is a necessary precondition for the separation. Thus, the ambiguity of embodiment. Changes in organic materiality result in (or are expected to) altering subject-ivity and narratives from organ transplant recipients suggest that the organs they received from another human donor cause subject-ivity changes; a human source, the recipient narrates how she can take on characteristics from the donor incorporating their organ and attributes of their previous life. An organ from a pig placed into the body has the potential to contaminate not just the human body but the person, making the recipient like a pig (and there are beliefs about 'dirty pigs'). A preference for personalised organs, bioprinted from the person, is the preferred option and the safest as it avoids risks to subjectivity alteration from organic contamination (Sanner 2001a). These stories of the organ are important in producing vari-able effects in embodiment. Then different kinds of organic sources are believed to cause various changes to the human body and, sub-sequently, the person. This is not the case when it comes to different types of materiality, as is the case with cybernetic technology.

The everyday cyborg is uniquely embodied as a hybrid of cyber-netic and organism, and there are multiple layers of vulnerabil-ities associated with the new body condition ranging from when the device is implanted and causing alienation (felt when the integrity of the body is breached and when it disrupts the body image). Indeed, in the case of ICDs, the technology is neither vis-ible nor invisible but remains present. The ICD is an alien presence experienced by some everyday cyborgs as a presence and altering their relationships with others (and indeed affecting the relations that others have with the everyday cyborg). As discussed earlier in Chapter 2, survey recipients claimed not to want a mechanical implant as it was perceived as being unnatural and uncomfortable. Such technological additions do not appear to alter subjectivity in the way that human or non-human animal transplants do. The machine is a different type of material that never came from a living being. It was made by a human but never came from a human. The cybernetic technology is not fleshy and has no previous association with any living being. There is no risk, therefore, of contamination of characteristics from the source. Technologies such as ICDs have been made and manufactured and have no association with living a previous life.

C3I functioning

The device's proximity into the body brings with it a remoteness and lack of accessibility, cementing the vulnerabilities caused by lack of choice to become cyborg by the inaccessibility of the cybernetic device. Its alien presence is felt on many occasions after implantation, mainly when it activates a discharge of shocks, leading to an unsettling question of who is in charge, or control of the everyday cyborg's body. Cybernetic systems are closed-loop systems that control aspects of the individual's physiological processes. It raises the possibilities that technology can and does go wrong – in the survey reported in Chapter 2, those preferring not to have a mechanical implant related it to ideas about reliable functioning whereby machines, break, rust and malfunction; 'technology and machines break more often than natural things'. Previous research with ICD patients confirms that inappropriate shocks do happen and cardiac devices have been the subject of recalls in recent years.

Nevertheless, the risks to the everyday cyborg stem not only from the ICD malfunctioning but carrying out the process that it was implanted into the cyborg body for – that is, to discharge electrical shocks to stop the heart going into a life-threatening arrhythmia. How such vulnerabilities are dealt with relating to implantation, subsequent cyborgisation and activation will be turned to in the next chapter when I focus upon what life is like as an everyday cyborg, as related by them. In Chapter 4, I give voice to the everyday cyborgs about their own experiences of cyborgisation through the implantation of an ICD.

Notes

1 https://en.wikipedia.org/wiki/Neil_Harbisson (accessed January 2020).
2 When a robot 'humanises' as in the film 'Bicentennial Man' (1999) – he does so to the point that when he feels emotions and forms relationships, he suffers emotional angst about the meaning (and ending) of life.
3 The relationship between fiction and non-fiction became closer when researchers at Osaka University in China introduced 'Geminoid F', an android unable to walk but capable of eye contact and described by her fans as the 'world's sexiest robot', see: www.cbc.ca/news/trending/world-s-sexiest-robot-causes-a-frenzy-at-beijing-tech-conference-1.3340974 (accessed November 2018).
4 www2.warwick.ac.uk/fac/med/research/hsri/emergencycare/prehospitalcare/jrcalcstakeholderwebsite/guidelines/the_implantable_cardioverter_defibrillator_icd_2006.pdf (accessed February 2020).
5 www.nhlbi.nih.gov/health/educational/hearttruth/index.htm. (accessed March 2020).
6 It was not until 2015 that the SynCardia Total Artificial Heart was modified and made smaller for women, see: www.sciencedaily.com/releases/2015/07/150701140901.htm (accessed November 2018).
7 Generally, such studies utilise survey methodologies of standard closed format questionnaires (Irvine, Dorian and Baker, 2002, Sears and Conti, 2003, Francis, Johnson and Niehaus, 2006, Kuhl et al., 2006).
8 www2.warwick.ac.uk/fac/med/research/hsri/emergencycare/prehospitalcare/jrcalcstakeholderwebsite/guidelines/the_implantable_cardioverter_defibrillator_icd_2006.pdf (accessed May 2019).
9 www.sciencemag.org/news/2015/02/could-wireless-pacemaker-let-hackers-take-control-your-heart (accessed March 2019).
10 www.medtronic.com/se-sv/healthcare-professionals/products/cardiac-rhythm/patient-management-carelink/medtronic-carelink-network-cardiac-device-patients.html (accessed October 2008).
11 www.aami.org/newsviews/newsdetail.aspx?ItemNumber=6475 (accessed February 2020).

4

Everyday cyborgs and the love-hate cybernetic relationship

Introduction

The term cyborg rarely appears in the sociology of health or medicine literature and seems never used about people who live with techno-logical modifications as a form of therapy. This is a curious absence (the absence itself rarely commented upon) given the increasing reli-ance on cybernetic technologies by Western medical professionals in economically developed societies. Reluctance to use the term cyborg more generally is related to the widespread knowledge of the cyborg *in extremis*; the inhumane, often male, monsters depicted in modern science-fiction, horror and popular media. They lose their human identity via a loss of humanity through the additions of cybernetic biotechnologies to their human forms (Oetler, 1995). The term cyborg, as discussed in the last chapter, however, was first introduced in the 1960s, predicting a need for closed-loop feedback mechanisms to regulate body responses during future space travel (Clynes and Kline, 1960). Such technological modifications did not change the male space traveller. Science and technology scholars and feminists reinvigorated the cyborg, and Donna Haraway's influ-ential conceptualisation of the cyborg is of a liberating figure that is ahistorical and post-gender, which is why it can offer an ability to liberate from classificatory dualist categories (1991). As I shall outline in this chapter, the everyday versions of the cyborg have little in common with the science-fiction cyborg apart from being male living as a techno-organic hybridity. Then everyday cyborgs are modified but not enhanced by their technological modifications; their emotions and feelings are not suppressed but heightened. As most psychological studies conducted with ICD patients show, there is a high prevalence of anxiety, depression and even anger in the ICD population. ICDs can cause cyborgs and their significant others emotional, physiological, psychological and social challenges that are rarely made visible. A cyborg individual or cyborg group identification thus reawakens interest in the techno-organic hybrid condition leading to new understandings about the obstacles as well as the benefits that implants pose.

By identifying and defining the everyday cyborg population, we begin to see how it affects the individual and their significant others. Re-appropriating the term cyborg for the everyday, as I will go on to show, reinserts issues about: what cyborgs need to live happy and fulfilling lives; what kind of support they and their significant others might find useful; as well as what type of information and understanding is required to acclimatise to a new techno-organic coalition. At the very minimum, the ICD offers a safety net, an umbrella to shelter them from death by SCA. This dependency invokes new vulnerabilities, as ICD and other implantable medical technologies are often out of reach of immediate human intervention and control. Becoming cyborg and an essential part of the cyborgisation process is not about changing subjectivity through the alteration of materiality that organic transplants cause through contamination. Unlike contamination reported from organic hybrids in previous chapters, the techno-organic hybrids experience technological invasion and device alienation. Then specific obstacles to the everyday cyborgs relate acclimatisation to a new hybridity that is initially alienating. Acclimatisation is a process whereby the ICD, experienced as an alien invader, becomes a part of their lives and their body. For everyday cyborgs with ICDs, their lives depend on the technology's autonomous *functioning* and this may be just as much a challenge as the ICD malfunctioning.

Finding and talking with the everyday cyborgs

I set out to find and talk with the everyday cyborgs. To me, it appeared crucial that the story of the ICD and cyborgisation had to be told from the cyborg's standpoint. To do so, I required the assistance of those involved in their creation and follow-up. In 2014, this research with everyday ICD cyborgs and significant others gained NHS ethical approvals, and participants were recruited using NHS gatekeepers through a consent-to-consent approach. Cardiac surgeons and electrophysiologists who create and maintain the everyday cyborgs identified and approached them on my behalf with information about the study and a consent form to return to me. I have no way of telling, therefore, which everyday cyborgs were approached by them and which refused to take part in this study. Of the 21 that agreed to participate, four everyday cyborgs were 'new', having received their ICDs in the six months before being interviewed. All of the new everyday cyborgs agreed to a repeat interview after a year, so that we could reflect on their experiences. This strategy offered a reflection on the accounts they had given a year previously, and also an updated one on what had changed in their life. These 'then and now' accounts they had given could be compared to the accounts of the older everyday ICD cyborgs when talking about their periods of transition to a cyborg life. A few of the older generation everyday cyborgs were now living with their second ICD system as the devices are replaced after approximately eight years depending on their activity levels. These older everyday cyborgs had lived a techno-organic hybrid existence for many years; some were living longer as an everyday cyborg than as a non-cyborg human.

I met with the 21 everyday cyborgs who agreed to take part in interviews. Interviews usually took place at their home but sometimes in a café or at the hospital after routine clinic check-ups. Before the meeting, I suggested they might want to invite others to be present and sent an additional consent form to give to them and sign. This invitation served the purpose of offering extra support when talking about the cyborgisation process, and if they felt inclined, they could share their thoughts and experiences. Wives, husbands or partners joined in 13 of the interviews, having completed an additional consent form. Occasionally, daughters, sons-in-law and grandchildren were present and contributed to the narratives. Generally, the presence of another person was supportive and helped the everyday cyborg recollection of events and enriched them with their perspective. However, it may have affected what the everyday cyborg was prepared to say in front of others – this appeared to be the case, for example, in Ramsay's interview when his wife Fay was present as I will show later.

Interviews were generally open-ended and flexible and could last from an hour to three hours. In the discussion, we covered areas such as: the circumstances up to and including the decision to implant the ICD; the experience of having one implanted; challenges and benefits of ICDs as well as thoughts more generally, about how it had affected their life, including views of the ICD firing or not. In some cases, we ended with discussing whether they would want or had thought about the removal of the ICD. Broaching death, dying and the ICD was extremely difficult and I erred on the side of caution by not raising it unless I was sure it would not upset anyone. Interestingly, this may be a reason why only a few of the everyday cyborgs recalled having a conversation with a health professional about removal as I go on to discuss later. That is, because they may have attempted to avoid unnecessarily upsetting the everyday cyborg.

Interviews were recorded, transcribed verbatim and then analysed, influenced by grounded theory and using an iterative approach to organising the transcripts, generating the codes, analysing the coding, and comparing themes in and between the coding sections of the interviews. This process was aided with the usage of the software package Nvivo 11. In the following accounts, I have kept as per participant wishes, their first names or a pseudonym they suggest. I have chosen to keep the Scottish vernacular and phrases in the quotes I use because, as I have emphasised, these are their stories and therefore should be told in their way and their own words.

Naming the cyborg?

During the interviews, I did not specifically ask the participants whether they identified themselves as a cyborg or not. This was for numerous reasons. Partly, the frequent equation of cyborgs (organic-technological hybrids) with androids (robots in human form) and robots (no organic or living parts) made it difficult to tell what exactly was being referred to (e.g. in the survey results there appeared to be little distinction being drawn by the respondents). The cultural baggage the term carries relating to the pervasiveness of the horror or science-fiction 'cyborg-as-monster' as I discussed in the previous chapters made it unlikely anyone would identify as such. Indeed, none of the everyday cyborgs apart from one mentioned the term 'cyborg' spontaneously to describe himself, and he thought it a description only he could use and was not to be used by others to describe him. Researching the term 'cyborg' made me realise that the conflation of the cyborg-as-monster with the everyday cyborg will be a significant and on-going issue.

This caused me to think carefully about what benefit using such a controversial term would offer, for example, discussing individual vulnerability as well as the stratification in cyborgisation as a form of 'cyborg sexism'.

Who are the everyday cyborgs?

Three everyday cyborgs were women, and 18 were men with ages ranging from 32 to 82 at the time of interview. This reflects the gender distribution of ICD implantation in the US and UK that is heavily weighted towards men. However, it does not follow (and nor would I claim) that the following findings are representative of all individuals; only that it appears to reflect general demographics regarding gender distribution.

Eleven had survived an SCA (see Table 4.1 below) and ten had suffered a heart attack and were thought likely to have a sudden cardiac episode. Some had genetic conditions that indicated they had a high risk of SCA, such as Brugada syndrome, arrhythmogenic right ventricular cardiomyopathy (ARVC), or Long-QT syndrome, and therefore were given an ICD for prophylactic reasons. For one or two of the individuals I interviewed, the cause of the sustained arrhythmias or arrest remained unknown. There appeared to be stress or 'heart-ache' in the family of the everyday cyborgs. There is on-going research into a condition called 'Takobutso Syndrome', or stress cardiomyopathy, that a person might experience after a devastating loss (although I am not suggesting that this was the case for these people who had an SCA with no explanation).

Eleven had reported never experiencing a shock. Six had been shocked once, and five had experienced shocks from their ICDs on several occasions. Two had received consecutive shocks, on the same occasion known as 'storms' (see Table 4.1 Demographics of everyday cyborgs). As I demonstrate, however, it was challenging to tally whether the ICD had fired or not with the experience of

Table 4.1 Demographics of everyday cyborgs

	Gender	Age group	Marital status	How long ICD	Firings	SCA
1 Alfred	Male	61–70	Married	over 5 yrs	Multiple	Yes
2 Audrey	Female	over 70	Married	under 6 mths	Once	Yes
3 David	Male	41–60	Relationship	over 5 yrs	Once*	Yes
4 Timothy	Male	over 70	Widowed	over 5 yrs	Multiple**	No
5 Graeme	Male	61–70	Married	over 5 yrs	None	Yes
6 Steven	Male	61–70	Relationship	over 5 yrs	Multiple**	Yes
7 Mark	Male	61–70	Married	under 6 mths	None	No
8 Jamie	Male	over 70	Married	over 5 yrs	Once	No
9 Luke	Male	over 70	Married	1–4 yrs	None	Yes
10 John	Male	61–70	Divorced	1–4 yrs	Once	No
11 Cathy	Female	41–60	Married	over 5 yrs	Once	Yes
12 Maggie	Female	under 40	Single	under 6 mths	None	No
13 Michael	Male	61–70	Married	over 5 yrs	None	Yes
14 Neil	Male	over 70	Divorced	over 5 yrs	Multiple	No
15 Shawn	Male	under 40	Relationship	over 5 yrs	Multiple*	No
16 Norman	Male	61–70	Married	over 5 yrs	None	Yes
17 Ramsay	Male	61–70	Married	over 5 yrs	None	Yes
18 Jason	Male	61–70	Married	over 5 yrs	None	Yes
19 Stella	Female	61–70	Married	under 6 mths	None	No
20 Stewart	Male	61–70	Married	over 5 yrs	None***	No
21 Thomas	Male	41–60	Married	1–4 yrs	None	No

*Said to be inappropriate
**Consecutively known as a 'storm'
***it was not clear whether Stewart had received shocks or cardioversion or indeed, both

the everyday cyborg. That is, there were cases where the everyday cyborg had experienced a shock, but the ICD had not recorded it (a 'phantom shock') or occasions when the ICD had fired, but the everyday cyborg had not been aware of it.

The broken hearts

Most had had a specific event or incident relating to their heart. However, others, as I said above, had had the ICD fitted for the prevention of an SCA despite not having experienced any type of cardiac episode (Maggie and Timothy). Attempting to assess whether different experiences relating to the ICD had some association with the kind of cardiac event (failure, disease, attack, arrest or genetic probability of having an SCA) or not is challenging to tease out in such a small sample. Two individuals, Maggie and Timothy, appear to have had more problems than others in living their life with their heart device, for example, alienation at implantation and device activation. Maggie had not experienced an SCA, and Timothy had no recollection of having had one. Without warning, and while visiting a friend in the hospital, Timothy had lost consciousness, and the next thing he remembers was waking up with the ICD implanted. Maggie has the genetic condition ARVC which led to her having an ICD implanted prophylactically. At 32 years old, she was the youngest of the group and was also the 'newest' everyday cyborg having been recently implanted only six weeks earlier. She was a keen runner and had been training to run half marathons but this was no longer possible for her.

Heart attacks and SCAs

Although he had suffered his heart attack 20 years ago, Steven could vividly remember the circumstances of it. He recalled that he was having his hair cut when he felt a pain in his chest, accompanied by feelings of intense nausea and sweating. He managed to make his way home where he felt the pain then becoming unbearable, comparing it to an 'elephant standing on his chest'. He called an ambulance and had three consecutive heart attacks in the hospital. These heart attacks had caused the structural damage to Steven's heart that would, over the years, affect the heart's electrical impulses required for a steady-state heart rate, leading him to have an ICD implanted.

Mark was in his late 60s when I interviewed him and had worked as a servitor at a university. He reported how, over many years, his heart failure had gotten progressively worse, and indeed his heart was slowly failing him, and there was no cure. Mark told me: 'It was getting worse and worse with the breathing that I was putting my socks and pants and that on by numbers, 1, 2, 3 go ...' The ICD he had implanted had pacing abilities as well as a defibrillator and he believed the pacing element helped his breathing.

Eleven of the everyday cyborgs I interviewed had survived an SCA. Cathy was 43 years old, and a police officer when I met with her and her husband. She had previously been diagnosed with Long-QT syndrome, however, her arrhythmias she believed were being well controlled with the use of beta-blockers. Then she recalled 'blacking out' at work during a physical training exercise:

> **Cathy:** Luckily, there was a PC who was a nurse in her former life was there, and they were about to perform CPR on me because I'd gone blue when I came to. I remember hearing voices, but everything still being dark at that point, and it was almost like I was frightened to open my eyes to see what was going on, but I couldn't. Again, it could probably only have been a matter of seconds, but for me, it felt a while.

Cathy was one of only a few everyday cyborgs able to return to work, albeit on desk duties after her ICD was implanted. Happily, Cathy and her husband became parents to twin daughters, and the ICD had little effect on the pregnancy.

Five years previously, Ramsay suffered an SCA at his mother-in-law's funeral. Previously he had been in robust health with no health conditions or indications of any heart problems. He would not have survived the SCA if it wasn't for his wife's sister, who was a nurse, administering CPR. Ramsay remembered little of the incident. He has changed since, however, as his wife Fay recalled during our interview:

> **Fay:** He's not the same person as what he was before he had that.
> **Gill:** In what way, do you think?

Fay: His mood swings. His temperament now, he's, he is not the same person.

Later, when Ramsay had left the room, she added:

> **Fay:** He [Ramsay] never used to like being left on his own, like, well, him, he wouldn't be able to watch Aidan [grand-son] to start with either, on his own [after ICD implantation]. Whereas before it, it [SCA] happened, he used to watch him. But no, he's a bit anxious now. If, if he's left for too long, I think, on his own.

Previous studies have discussed the anger, anxiety and depression that can result from either a heart condition or living with an ICD. However, it was unclear which had had the most significant effect. Ramsay suggests it was to do with losing his job:

> **Ramsay:** Aye. I think it's just frustration of not being working, honestly.
> **Gill:** Do you?
> **Ramsay:** I think so; honestly, I think that's what it is.
> **Gill:** Right. So it's not anything to do with, it's not anything to do with the, the cardiac arrest ...
> **Ramsay:** I don't think so.
> **Gill:** ... or having the defibrillator, or anything like that?
> **Ramsay:** No, no, honestly that doesnae bother me, eh.

For Ramsay, the source of his frustration was based on his inability to return to his work in the building trade which gave him a sense of purpose as a 'bread-winner,' and he appeared to have had a strong male circle of friends and acquaintances. His tentative answer ('I don't think so') that it was not the SCA that had changed his identity suggests there was more to the effects of the SCA than Ramsay would admit in the presence of his wife. Ramsay, like other everyday cyborgs in this study (and in studies with cardiac patients discussed in the last chapter), can, as Charmaz has described: 'Chronic illness assaults the body and threatens the integrity of self" (1995: 657). Further, 'ill people adapt when they try to accommodate and flow with the experience of illness' (1995: 67). Ramsay may still be adjusting; his wife Fay suggested that 'he wouldn't be able to watch Aidan to start with', implying that he could do so now.

Outside-in: cyborgisation will be televised

The creation of an everyday cyborg is a relatively fast and visually unique experience in which the patient is conscious and aware throughout the procedure. A local anaesthetic is used as it is beneficial, 'in terms of procedural cost, duration and safety in patients' (Lipscomb, Linker and Fitzpatrick, 1998: 255). The procedure to insert the ICD system takes a matter of hours in an operating theatre (OT). The cardiac surgeon, supported by a team makes a 5 cm opening in the left-hand side of the chest (akin to where the top pocket of a jacket might sit). The ICD wires are manoeuvred from the chest incision, into the atrium of the heart and the ventricle, before the generator is placed into the pectoral chest. A representative of the ICD manufacturer is present during the procedure to advise on the use of the hardware, for example, the thickness of wires. Guiding the wires into the chambers of the heart requires the cardiologist to have significant levels of skill and patience attempting to do this when the heart is beating. Indeed, as reported in the last chapter, ICD manufacturer Medtronic voluntarily recalled their devices that had thinner 'sprint fidelis' leads as making the wires thinner to aid the process of implantation entering into the heart was predicted to lead to potentially higher mortality rates (Ellenbogen, Wood and Swerdlow, 2008).

The soon-to-be everyday cyborgs have their faces partially covered so that they cannot see what the surgeon is doing to their body, but they can observe the progress above their head on two monitors. As Mark wryly commented when recalling details of the procedure, 'I never knew it was all done on the telly.' For some the visualisation was enriching, as Alfred related:

> Alfred: So, to, that was a positive and as I say, I found the actual receiving it quite an interesting exercise, because you're really quite awake, apart from the local injection on your chest and your throat because they would have to break into your vein to get into your arm. You're watching all this on … and, watch them screw the wire into your heart.

Different reflective surfaces and mirrors in the OT also offered an alternative visual experience to some of the patients during the procedure:

Maggie: ... well, I suppose it's a light, it must be one of these big lights that you can pull down, but it's, like, mirrored, it's, like, reflective. And I could ... so I could see. So, I saw them making the incision, and I could see, um, like, my muscle, and I could see, like, a little bit of fat. And I was saying, 'is that fat?', 'is that fat?', 'why is there fat there?' [Laugh]

Glimpses of the inside of their body was a unique and fascinating experience for a few. The visual experience of watching the wires being carefully threaded and pushed into the everyday cyborg's body is simultaneously experienced on the monitors while occurring in their bodies; they can see into the muscle and as Maggie asks 'is that fat?'

Other everyday cyborgs found the insertion uncomfortable. Stella, despite being heavily sedated, recalled that the procedure had painful moments. She remembered telling the cardiologist: 'I can feel you cutting me ... like something stinging' and that how 'at that point they [operating theatre staff] just pumped, pumped more in, the sedative or something, whatever they give you'. This incision can constitute a painful breach as the first stage of the implantation for the patient as feeding the wires into the heart is a challenge for the surgeon.

One of the last phases is placing the battery and the generator into the cavity of the chest. Internally, the body is tightly packed with organs, and there is little extra room for adding an ICD despite it being roughly the size of a matchbox. Both Ian and Michael remarked on how painful this aspect of the procedure was for them:

Ian: ... as if I was going to go right through the trolley. I mean he apologised again like for pressing so hard, it was to get this. I couldn't visualise as to what it even looked like. I was very surprised when ... I mean it's just a, it's just a box.

Ian's wife: And it says a lot for them [surgical team] too because they're ... I mean, they're human beings. I know it's their job, but it must affect them but they must be able to shut off after they've done their job, but they must ... I mean, they know they're inflicting pain on you but it's for your own good, you know.

Ian seemed surprised about the actual size of the ICD – 'it's just a box' – which appears to indicate that, based on his experience of the device's implantation, the ICD felt more substantial than it was. Ian's wife was quite philosophical about Ian's experience, commenting on the ability of those present in the OT to disassociate in order to continue with the procedure. Michael found his first ICD implantation very painful:

> **Michael:** It's all over with me, I've been through so much pain in my life it doesn't really matter. I don't know why it was so painful, but they seemed to keep pushing and pushing into my shoulder blade. I said, 'no, I can't put up with much more of this'. 'I'll give you some more relief', he said. I don't know what they did, but they gave me some more relief, but that didn't work, then all of a sudden this guy kept pressing, and I just passed out from the pain. I couldn't put up with it, it was horrible, one of my worst experiences. But then when I saw that this thing, it was like a matchbox, that's why I suppose they're [ICDs] flat now.

Michael was understandably anxious when he had to have his ICD replaced due to the depletion of its battery. His concerns proved to be misplaced as the second time Michael said he was in 'fairyland' and did not recall any discomfort whatsoever. Indeed, a study conducted in 1998 reviewed 33 patients' experiences after having an ICD implanted using local anaesthetic and sedation, and found that almost none recalled the procedure, although one reported awareness of 'pushing'. Seven suggested the process was painless but recalled a test shock reporting either awareness or discomfort with the shock (Lipscomb, Linker and Fitzpatrick, 1998). None of the everyday cyborgs in this study reported experiencing a test shock – when the ICD is implanted the shock discharge can be tested to ensure the ICD will work at the heart rate threshold that has been set for the individual.

Although patients like Stella mentioned above, found the incision the most painful assault on the skin, others reported that the surgeon's attempts to find a space for the ICD in the chest was extremely uncomfortable. The placing of the ICD generator into the chest cavity requires the surgeon to use some force and can be a difficult experience for both the surgeon and the everyday cyborg. There is little space inside most human organs, apart from the lungs, stomach and inner ear canals. Unlike organ transplantation where the organ is often removed (exceptions being in the case of kidney transplantation), anything that is added to an already full viscera space will protrude. As a result, the ICD causes a bulging from under the skin and is a permanent silhouette on the skin of the chest. A few participants reported that the outline could be troubling for them, and Timothy admitted to having never really got used to having the ICD in his body. He related how 'your body shouldn't have a square lump like that'. The placing of the ICD leaves a scar and an imprint, a silhouette on the skin, marking where the intrusion occurred and where the body's integrity has been breached. The ICD is very noticeable in the few weeks after surgery and at times after that, where the skin silhouette acts as a continual reminder of the presence of a cybernetic system. In Leder's terms, the ICD is causing the body to become an 'absent absence' (1990) as shown in John's comments:

> **John:** And it's almost like ... and I don't want, I don't want to be ... it's a bit like being continually reminded that you've got this condition. I mean, in some respects I would rather just blend into society and just become an ordinary person again, you know.
>
> **Gill:** Do you not think you're an ordinary person?
>
> **John:** Well, I feel I'm, to some extent I feel extraordinary because I feel ...
>
> **Gill:** Extraordinary. [Laughing]
>
> **John:** ... I'm being kept, I'm being kept alive by that, you know.

The silhouette of cybernetic technology is a reminder of the everyday cyborg's mortality. The daily routine 'absence' of the body was no longer absent; the body and especially the scarification and silhouette caused by the ICD on the chest resulted in a heightened awareness of it causing what Leder (1990) calls a 'dys-appearance'. Notably, there is no subjectivity alteration said to occur at this point as is the case of organic human or non-human animal transplants.

Inside out: an absent absence

The rehabilitation for most everyday cyborgs did not have adverse or damaging consequences. This is not to say that it was not challenging and frequently mentioned was the on-going unwelcome presence of the ICD in the body. It is a tangible sensation both through sight and touch, but its presence constitutes more than sensory perception. In regular interaction, Leder suggests different regions of the body 'recede' from direct experience and therefore constitute an absence (1990). Our absent bodies are a daily aspect of everyday living, and it is only at times of bodily change or pain that our body becomes present. Such body modification, as in the case of ICD implantation, causes the 'absent absence' and a 'dys-appearance' (Leder, 1990), meaning that absent bodies are no longer absent.

For some, the feeling of the ICDs causing an 'absent absence' inside their body was particularly acute in the weeks that followed the surgery. From inside the body, the feeling of the ICD's presence was there variously when showering, lying down or sleeping on the left side where the ICD was placed. This meant that initially at least, the everyday cyborg had to alter their posture and their body's usual resting position. Audrey said: 'I can't sleep on that side [where the ICD is], I have to sleep on my back or on my other side.' Stella suggested a similar experience: 'I can feel it, sometimes, if I'm lying down, it'll jut out a bit more and I'll go … (makes a movement to push it back).' Alfred suggested:

> Well, I'm really quite thankful because I mean it's saved my life bloody three times. But, it is a bit of an inconvenience, because it does stick up and, you know, you can, when you're sleeping, it kind of interferes if you're on one side.

The ICD is a foreign device and to some constitutes an alien invasion creating an absent absence in that part of the body. For Jason, he related to me how: 'I felt that you … you were conscious of it being there all the time'. The newest and youngest of the everyday cyborgs, Maggie, who had her ICD implanted six weeks previous to our interview, was initially concerned about how her everyday movements might affect the positioning of the ICD:

> I wasn't moving my arm really, but yeah, I was … er, the first initially … yeah, yeah, I was really worried about, um, you know, lifting things up and the wires dislodging. Which I now understand is actually really pretty difficult.

In a conversation we were having about her sister's pregnancy, Maggie drew out the differences between them:

> **Maggie:** … you know, whatever. Um and again, you know, they can help the … turn the baby around and get the baby out and what

not. But it … like, to put a machine, um, something that's not nat-ural to keep you alive, I'm not sure that I'm totally 100 per cent convinced, even though I've got one. [Laugh] You know, and since I got it implanted, I've thought about it even more.

Maggie had difficulties accepting the ICD because, to her, it was a machine and was therefore 'unnatural'. Her statement that 'I thought about it [ICD] even more' demonstrates how an 'absent absence' of the ICD is a presence in the lives of everyday cyborgs. The daily routine 'absence' of the body was no longer absent; the body, and especially the scarification and silhouette caused by the ICD on the chest, resulted in a heightened awareness of it. Jason discussed how difficult an 'absent absence' is and the feelings that resulted:

> **Jason:** … once that got fitted in there, I wanted to tear it back out again. I did … I was quite … I … I don't know what the word was, but I just didn't like it in there …
>
> **Gill:** No.
>
> **Jason:** I didn't want it.

Cyborgisation incurs emotional costs and creates disturbing thoughts. Although Jason eventually acclimatised to his ICD, he reported initially being 'more thingmied (scots slang for "agitated" or "flustered") about the ICD as I was about the blooming triple bypass operation, believe it or not.' When probed on why this was the case, he suggested, 'Just the thought of it [ICD] being there. Aye, that's all it was.' Hence, although I have emphasised the importance of placing the everyday cyborg's voice and vernacular at the centre of the story about the cyborgisation process, there are, for some, no words that can describe the various thoughts and feelings it causes. There is no vocabulary or lexicon readily available to describe this condition of neither being sick nor well – that is, not a disease or illness – but neither are they in an altogether healthy state, so per-haps better described as an 'un-health'.

See me; feel me

Most everyday cyborgs were discharged from the hospital within a day or two although recovery could take much longer. This has implications for the economic independence that breadwinners such as Ramsay, above, mentions as finding frustrating. The consequence for some could be particularly harsh. Thomas, like Ramsay, worked in the trades. He was a plumber until he lost his job:

> **Thomas:** Mm. I ... I was ... well, I do feel I was a bit ... I don't know if it's anxiety or depression or anything, but after I got it done because I was off my work ...
>
> **Gill:** When, er, the device got fitted?
>
> **Thomas:** Aye and then, I ... they said about six weeks [was needed for recovery], and then I used all my savings to keep the house going and then ... So I ... I ... I claimed house insurance and they said, you never declared you had a heart condition. I said, look at my last mortgage ... my last mortgage, but, er, I lost ... well, I ended up ... had to go bankrupt. I lost my house. Everything.

'He lost everything'. Thomas lost his job as a trade plumber and his house, leading him to file for bankruptcy. Thankfully such consequences were infrequently reported during interviews, although the loss of employment was a common theme in all of them. It is difficult to tell whether the loss of employment has to do with the physical limitations or the restrictions on driving that follows the ICD implantation. For some, however, it was clear that their lives were irreversibly altered and they needed to adjust. To accomplish this adjustment and acclimatisation, they employed strategies to balance what they had lost, against what they had gained (as discussed below).

Acclimatisation and sinking

The ICD constitutes, for most everyday cyborgs, a presence, an irony when absence that is absent, or in Leder's terms, a 'dys-appearance' (Leder, 1990). Sobchack (2010) writes of how this dys-appearance plays out in terms of amputation and of prosthetics. She expands on Leder's dys-appearance by noting that 'what is physically absent and what is ostensibly artificial can be – and often are – more experientially present or embodied than birthed, intact, or residual limbs'

(Sobchack, 2010). The ICD device breaches the body integrity and image and is more present; it is straddling the body boundaries of inside-out and outside-in and through its placement, causing the absence of that particular body site to become present. Just as it can be even more present, then so it can be less present in experiential terms. It is a process that is fluid and subject to change over time. It is the case, as Dalibert observes in her research with patients who have a deep brain stimulator, that the device is 'under the skin [and] amounts neither to ... disappearance nor to its transparency but rather entails new body-technology configurations and ways of being in the world' (2016: 216).

For some, the 'absent absence' issue was never an issue to begin with. Stewart suggested that, although he was conscious of his ICD catching on clothing, it did not concern him. Jokingly, he remarked: 'Luckily I don't wear a bra [laughter].' Three of the four everyday cyborgs were women, and there was some mention of concern about body image, but for Stella: 'No. You wouldn't know it was there until, I mean, unless you saw this wee bit sticking out.' Both Stewart and Stella did not report any concerns at all about their ICD and felt the benefit from it – as I shall cover later, their ICD journeys were not beset with some of the challenges that others had. Although an ICD would settle into the body, overcoming dys-appearance took variable amounts of time and different strategies.

From alien invasion to part-of-me

The new 'body-technology' configuration that Dalibert (2016) refers to can involve a level of incorporation (De Preester and Tsakiris, 2009) or acclimatisation (Haddow, Harmon and Gilman, 2015). In the case of the ICD, the dys-appearance is resolved through a process of acclimatisation. This involves the ICD becoming a part of the body, and no longer an alien presence. For example, researchers argue that prosthetic users are encouraged to view their prosthesis as a 'corporeal structure' that is more than a tool like a cane or walking stick (Murray, 2004). De Preester and Tsakiris draw upon an account given by a man who was born without a foot (quoted in Murray, 2004):

> One of the major factors in my satisfaction with a new prosthesis is how little I feel it. That may sound strange, but to me, my prosthesis is an extension of my body. (I can actually 'feel' some things that come into contact with it, without having to see them … It must 'feel' as close to not being there as possible.)
>
> (Murray, 2004: 970 quoted in De Preester and Tsakiris, 2009: 310)

Like the interviewee in Murray's study, when I talked with Maggie roughly ten months after our first interview, she described how her relation to her ICD had changed from its initial alienating presence:

> **Maggie:** There's … yeah, 'cause as in, basically, if I was to try … if you think about it in the opposite sense, if something happens to my body, the wires … you know, the wires do something. And it is, it's part. So, of course, maybe in, like, fifteen years or ten years' time, I will actually feel, you know, this is … *it is part of me*. And I suppose, in a way, maybe, you know, you might accept that it's … it's strange to think of accepting a piece of machinery that, sort of, is …
>
> (emphasis added)

Moreover, Neil drew an interesting analogy between his body and that of a ship:

> **Neil:** … was that when the device first goes in, it's, kind of like, a, kind of … it's more of a foreign body, if you like, to your … your system … and then once it had been in a long time, it, kind of … the wires and everything else that's there, kind of, get covered in all the, sort of, gunk that goes round your body and it becomes less and less of a, kind of, foreign body over time, because it … you know … you know, I suppose like a ship in the sea, it gets covered … you know, like …
>
> **Gill:** Barnacles?
>
> **Neil:** … it gets covered in barnacles and all these type things …

Neil suggests that the ICD undergoes a physical transformation as it gradually becomes coated in the 'gunk' of the organic body and therefore becomes less 'foreign'. Audrey described the ICD as 'being absorbed' into her body. John discusses how his ICD became physically less prominent:

> **John:** I mean, I mean I was obviously aware of it [ICD] being there.

Gill: Were you, uh-huh?

John: And in fact, I think I've put another half an, half an inch of fat over here since then.

Gill: [Laughing]

John: But when I got it, it seemed actually more prominent than it is just now.

Over time the ICD and its silhouette on the body becomes an absence again that characterises much of the relationship we have with our body in everyday life. We manage to not pay attention to the status of our bodies or indeed, our relationship with them and therefore are able to get on with our day-to-day living. What is perhaps remarkable is that for most, the ICD quickly and easily becomes part of the body and more significantly, part of the person. Stella had received a specialised ICD called a CRT-D to treat her heart failure, a device that is implanted with an additional wire around the back of the heart to coordinate a more efficient heartbeat. She told me that she 'instantly felt the benefit from it, if I didn't have it [ICD], I wouldn't be able to breathe, you know'. She readily suggested, 'it's *just part of me now*, it's no big deal'. For Stella, her ICD allowed her to breathe and gave her her previous life back. Stewart reported that his ICD was, 'You know. It's like my shoes. You know, I don't consider my shoes alien. I don't, I mean it's, obviously I wasn't born with it, *but it lets me be who I am*' (emphasis added). The turning point for Jason coming to accept his ICD was when the life-saving benefit of the ICD was explained:

> **Jason:** I did, aye. I wanted it out ... I told ... I asked them [medical professionals] that when I went up. And I got a bollocking, of course. [Laugh] And of course, the ... the nurse ... the ... the ... the lady said to me, she said right away, she says, well, Mr Campbell, she says, I'll tell you the truth, somebody had theirs in there for about years, just the same as you and they says ... but ... what the ... if ... if they didn't have had it in there, but a couple of month after it, er, the thing took a ... a ... a ... a ... it fired ...
>
> **Jason's wife:** Uhm-hmm.
>
> **Jason:** ... and saved the bloke's life ...
>
> **Gill:** Right. Uhm-hmm.

> Jason: ... and of course, ever since then, I've really said to myself, well, it's there for a reason really ... So I've been a wee bit more ... knowing ... I wasn't going to say happier, but I'm a wee bit more relaxed to the situation now and ...
>
> Jason's wife: Uhm-hmm. Time heals, doesn't it?

The acclimatisation to new hybridity for Jason was a process initially hindered by not experiencing the benefits of the cyborg life. However, time does heal, as Jason's wife remarked, in terms of a new comfortable synergy between the ICD (cyb) and the body (org).

For others, like David, if time was not a healer, then therapy certainly was. David was one of the oldest everyday cyborgs, and he had been fitted with his ICD 20 years previously. His accounts of his early experiences are similar to those that were shared by Jason. David related how it had stopped him 'sleeping, it was making me anxious ... it just had changed my body a bit and, I ... I felt it *wasn't part of me in* that it was a machine'. He offered a retrospective view of the way his relationship to the ICD changed over the years:

> David: ... when I first had this implanted, I, you know, it felt very much like my enemy, despite the fact that it could potentially save my life. Um and by the end of this long journey, I feel that ... I would feel very strange, without it, you know ... and so, um, I feel it has ... it has really *become part of me* in a way that I didn't ever expect it would.
>
> (emphasis added)

It was not until he had sought therapy that his relationship to the ICD had changed. Indeed, current guidance by the National Institute of Clinical Excellence in the UK has suggested that approximately 5 per cent of patients with an ICD need cognitive behavioural therapy after implantation (NICE, 2014: 40–41). However, this appears only to be a recommendation and is not widely available in the UK despite the variability in the way that acclimatisation to the alienation reported since implantation is resolved. For the everyday cyborgs, Maggie, Jason, David and Timothy, who reported issues with the ICD causing a bodily absent absence, they did not necessarily experience the benefit of the device. On the contrary, it could signify the life they had previously but had no longer. Then the process of acclimatisation and the ICD can be facilitated when the benefits of the ICD is experienced; it becomes a comfortable part of the body and a 'part of me'.

Others: protecting the ICD from others

Despite the ICD transformation from alien presence to a part of the body and 'part of me', it still required protection from the unexpected physical movements of other people. The everyday cyborgs seek to protect the ICD hardware from accidental damage by others. The unpredictability of other people's movements became important because the ICD is sitting inside the body but not far enough in as it was still noticeable from the outside. Then although it was far enough inside to be out of reach of the everyday cyborg, this did not mean that it felt safe and secure against blows or accidental damage from others. Perhaps partly due to its position as not being fully inside the body, it was thought to be at risk from others that could inadvertently damage the device:

> Luke's wife: My great-granddaughter will be eight this year and she comes up and torments him, he'll say go away because he's scared she would knock it.
> Gill: [turning to Luke] Do you think she would ...?
> Luke: I don't know if it would do any harm but I'm not taking the chance because she's so coarse ('heavy handed') the way she flings herself about.

The everyday cyborg's avoidance of physical contact was specific to the situation. It led to them avoiding certain individuals and environments that were deemed potentially damaging to the ICD, and perhaps by the association to the everyday cyborg. Jason was unable to visit the garage where he was previously employed due to some of the specific environmental restrictions such as avoiding arc welding, as well as being careful to avoid the physical demonstrativeness of his workmates:

> Jason: ... and when I went to my work, drivers were periodically ... or mechanics, they were putting their hands on the back of my shoulder like that and gripping me and they were

forgetting that I had ... And there was a lot of things like that and the garage itself ...

Jason's wife: Right in there, was about all his, sort of ...

Jason: ... had a lot of mechanical parts in there and it was all magnets and God knows what it was in there ... and I was dead scared to go in there in case the thing was going to set off and ...

Jason's wife: [Laugh]

Jason: ... it was terrible.

In terms of clinical guidance, everyday cyborgs are advised to avoid contact sports such as rugby, avoid magnets, airport and security devices, diathermy, MRI scanning and, in Jason's case, arc welding.

Check-ups: by significant others

The everyday cyborg might mostly be male, but he was not a 'Robocop' or even like the android 'Terminator'. On the contrary, he had the potential to suffer a cardiac event, and this resulted in over-protectiveness by the everyday cyborg's wife (or husband). Some like Ramsey and Jason clearly articulated how their masculine role as bread-winner had altered, for example. This led to tension in their close relationships. Fay, Ramsay's wife, recognises Ramsay might construe some of her behaviour as being 'overprotective' but she defended this by saying:

> **Fay:** Because he cracks up with me, Gill, because anywhere he goes, or when I'm away to my work or that, I'll phone him umpteen times a day. And he cracks up with me ... for god's sake, for god's sake! And I'll say, you werenae there that day, you didnae see what happened, ken.

She was witness to his SCA at her mother's funeral, and it was only due to her sister's intervention that Ramsay's life was saved. Then although her behaviour was viewed as being 'over-protective' and was complained about, it was entirely justified in Fay's view because she witnessed just how close Ramsay came to dying that day. The ICD was to protect the everyday cyborg from SCA; however, significant others saw their role now of protecting the everyday cyborg from themselves:

Mark's wife (on my second visit): It's a wee bit easier now, but at the start he wanted to go out and do things and he (Mark) just wasn't ... I mean I was terrified he would fall. I mean I only go to the wee shop and back again because I'm terrified in case he falls again. It's caused so much agro between us because he wants to do it and I'm saying to him, don't do it. Or will you please stay there till I come back? But, I mean, I get out on a Saturday, John [their son] takes him away a run [in the car] for the day.

Mark's wife: That's and then ... but of course one of the family came and sat with Mark until I came back.

Mark: Babysitting.

Understandably, for significant others, the implantation of an ICD was viewed with a tremendous sense of relief and gratitude. The ICD is intended to prevent an SCA occurring and indeed is so efficient that it will continue to shock the cyborg even when it is unnecessary to do so (as discussed further below regarding the circumstances of removal). The ICD can, therefore, be an additional layer of protection, watching along with those closest to the everyday cyborg. In some cases, it could allow them to step down from certain aspects of surveillance:

> **Stewart's wife:** ... when he (husband Stewart) was very ill I was concerned because you'd go to bed at night, this was before he had his ICD put in, we'd go to bed at night, and I'm listening to his breathing because sometimes ... it sounded as though he was going to stop. And then I thought, 'oh God, something's going on' and then he would breathe again. So, I really was, he was totally unaware of that because he was asleep ... So that I was very keen for him to have an ICD because I thought, well at least if I'm asleep and he stops breathing or whatever then something's going to happen to, to save him.

Loved ones and significant others were fully aware of the ICD's benefits and saw it as life insurance. In an exchange between Audrey and her husband Joseph, Audrey's ICD was explicitly referred to as 'life insurance':

> **Audrey:** Yes, I just ...
> **Joseph:** It's like having an insurance policy ...
> **Audrey:** ... take it for granted.

Joseph: ... you hope you never use it, but it ...
Audrey: Yes.
Joseph: ... it's good to know it's there.

Audrey was in her 80s when she received her ICD, and she believes that protests made by her daughters led to an overcoming of the initial reluctance to give her one. This may or may not be a reflection of the 'cyborg sexism' I discussed earlier when fewer women than men receive an ICD despite their propensity to suffer similar rates of heard conditions, albeit at an older age. The ICD is quite literally a form of life insurance and provides reassurance to significant others that they will not lose their loved one from an SCA. It does not mean that the significant others can stand down from their surveillance over their loved ones, however. Their loved ones still keep watch over the everyday cyborg to ensure they are not causing themselves any harm by what they see as potentially harmful behaviour, for example, by climbing ladders, which rather curiously was mentioned in several interviews.

Putting the ICD through its paces

For significant others, the ICD is 'on watch' from inside the bodies of everyday cyborgs, offering protection from an SCA through its C3I. The ICD can maintain close surveillance even when significant others are absent. However, the ICD itself requires check-ups, and hence the everyday cyborg is required to attend 'pacing clinics' for the device to be reviewed regarding battery depletion, evidence of cardioversion incidents or discharge of shocks:

Alfred: So, this type, I suppose it can pace your heart, speed it up or slow it down, but it can also cardiovert ...
Gill: Have you felt it pace? Have you felt it ever pace?
Alfred: I have had it happen to me in the clinic, because they speed it up and slow it down.
Gill: What does that feel like?
Alfred: It feels really odd, I have never really been aware of my heart very much, although some people are. So, having it speed up or slow down, you're very conscious as to ... but, you know, there's no reason for it to be done, it's not like

you've been running or something, so it's very strange, well, to me strange.

Stella echoed the odd sensation of her heart rate being slowed:

> **Stella:** They only put the wires on your legs, and where they usually put it, on the heart. But then they take your monitor thing, and they put it there. But then, they do all the things through the computer. And so she'll [electrophysiologist] say, 'I'm just gonna slow the heart'.
>
> **Gill:** She told you that?
>
> **Stella:** Aye.
>
> **Gill:** Uh-huh.
>
> **Stella:** And I think she done that a couple of times. But one of the times, I felt really woozy with it, and I was saying, oh I didn't feel right. And she just said, oh I'm sorry. And then, they did, you know, they click on the heart, and it just makes you feel all funny for a wee few seconds.

Remote monitoring

The ICD's surveillance functionality can be extended by exploiting the communication part of the C3I function for remote monitoring. Clinicians had given a couple of the everyday cyborgs in this research remote monitoring devices. These devices replace most of the clinic visits that the everyday cyborg undertakes every six months or so for a check-up (more frequently if the battery levels were depleting or if the device had fired). The upload of activity remotely from the ICD is scheduled with a date and time in advance, or as Stewart paraphrased it, he received a letter requesting him to 'plug yourself in'. Stella asked for a remote monitor when she was at the hospital clinic and was given one right away. 'It plugs in at the side of the bed. Lift it up, place it over the device, and it downloads everything,' said Stella. There are growing fears as discussed in the last chapter that hackers would be able to either interfere with the functioning of the device or capture data from it. When I asked Stella about the possibility of hackers using her data or accessing her device, she questioned the motivation of malicious intention, asking 'why someone would expend time, resources or energy in hacking her medical device?' As only a few of the everyday cyborgs had a remote monitoring unit, it is difficult to ascertain how common Stella's view was.

Generally, the remote unit is kept beside the bed. I asked Stewart if he knew why this was the case:

> Gill: I'm trying to think, why wouldn't they have it near you while, while, they wouldn't have something like during the day time that they would pick up an event, you know. Why is it like you say ...?
>
> Stewart: Because I'd be conscious then and I would know what was happening.
>
> Gill: So, at night?
>
> Stewart: Often, often my ... often my arrhythmias are, are at night. They're momentary, I mean they'll say, oh it only lasted, you know, nine-tenths of a second or something. But it's often and often just before you waken up in the morning.

While the cyborg sleeps, the sensory and communicative system of the ICD does not. What caused some concern from Stewart, however, as he humorously related, was that the medical profession could 'spy' on the everyday cyborg:

> Stewart: And she [electrophysiologist] said, she said, 'well your pace-maker[1] paced you and it didn't work and your pacemaker paced you again and it didn't work. And it charged up and it was just going to zap you and your heart sorted itself out.' [Laughs] But I found it's quite scary that she [electrophysiologist] can spy on me like that. [Laughs]

Essentially, the ICD can offer further surveillance for the medical experts into the patient's body even when the patient is not present in the clinic or even awake. This surveillance by clinicians is one whereby they can tell when the everyday cyborg is awake and active or at rest due to the activity level of the ICD. Unlike ten of the everyday cyborgs, Stewart had not received a shock and had an unproblematic relationship with his ICD. However, five of these ten had received shocks multiple times on the same occasion – an event known as a 'storm'. It is the narratives about shocks that I turn to next.

Reconciliation: shocking moments

Medical devices, such as ICDs, I have argued, can be considered cybernetic; defined as having a smart functionality fulfilling Haraway's C3I features, of command-control-communication-intelligence (1991). The cybernetic functionality takes the form of a feedback loop that senses a change in the environment, in this case, the heart's beat, and establishes an intervention to reinstate normality (through a series of small electric shocks to cardiovert) before assessing the success of it and possibly scaling up to shock the everyday cyborgs. The ICD can administer shocks up to 40 joules, which is much lower than an external defibrillator can (100–360j) but can still be painful for some.[2] Sometimes the shock can be given at least half a dozen times or more, before then recording and communicating the events either through remote monitoring or interrogation of the device at the clinic afterwards. For the everyday cyborg, a life-saving shock is an event that is not inevitable but is always possible. This possibility of shock may form a core part of the love/hate relationship the everyday cyborg had with their ICD.

Alfred's ICD had been implanted 11 years previously, and he experienced shocks on three separate occasions. Alfred's wife, Jean, said that when the ICD shocked Alfred the first time, she thought he was dying:

Jean: Alfred just as he described, you were just sitting there, and Alfred actually had a drink in his hand and that's what I noticed first, I just saw liquid splashing and I turned round, and at that point trying to think, well his eyes were rolling back in his head, and I thought he was dying, I thought that was it, so I grabbed the phone to get the paramedics. Then he suddenly came to and jumped up, and I said 'sit down,' and I think at the point I was thinking it could have been something to do with that.

Gill: To do with the ICD or to do with his heart?

Jean: The ICD, uh-huh or heart, just something not right there, so it was a bit of a shock.

As she says, without any irony, 'it was a bit of a shock'. Alfred tended to see his multiple experiences of non-consecutive shocks, that is, shocks which had occurred on separate occasions, as not being entirely unexpected; he had had a general feeling of malaise or being 'lightheaded' before the ICD went off. Alfred had received a university degree in physics to which he linked his pragmatic attitude towards the ICD:

> No, I think, I remember most of what happened, but I think I'm very pragmatic, you know, physics and stuff, so I tend to look at these things in a right factual sort of way, So, I knew I was in trouble, I knew they were wanting to give me something that would help it, so to me that was perfectly fine. The fact that I need to *walk about with a thing inside me seemed to me the ideal position I was* in, like if it was in your handbag and you left it at home sort of thing, you know, it's with you all the time. ... Anyway it all settled down so they let me go, and I guess at that point, you know, it's your first experience, and so it's doing what it says on the tin.
>
> (Alfred, emphasis added)

The ICD is doing 'exactly what it says on the tin.'

Pain and storms

Two everyday cyborgs experienced storms or consecutive firings within one period of time. Steven reported how he had been hung-over one day and this, he felt, had contributed to his ICD going off. Like Alfred, Steven had had some form of short-term awareness that his ICD was about to go off so like Albert, the shock did not come as a surprise, in that understanding of the word 'shock'. However, it had shocked him five times consecutively:

> **Steven's partner:** And, he was lying here and I looked at him and ... and he went, oh, here it's going again. And, h ... his body was just ...
> **Steven:** Boom.
> **Steven's partner:** ... jumping.
> **Gill:** Lifting? Right off the couch?
> **Steven:** Three times here, twice in the lift.
> **Steven's partner:** And, he was chalk white ...?
> **Steven:** But ... Aye, it's, er ...
> **Steven's partner:** But, as he says, it saved his life.

Understandably, Steven was keen to have the ICD removed after the ICD storm:

> **Steven:** And, er, I says to him, 'doctor, get this out of me'. I says, 'I canny go through that again'.
>
> **Gill:** Did you say that?
>
> **Steven:** Aye, I said that to him. I say, 'you better take this out' ... And, he stood there, and he says, 'look, that device probably saved your life'.

His ICD discharges a shock on one other occasion which he explained: 'Well ... It went off once, but that was my own fault ... I was trying to lift something awfully heavy.' After that, and with adjustments made to his medication, Steven did not suffer any further firing. In contrast, to these painful episodes, two everyday cyborgs said they were hardly aware that their ICD had gone off. Stewart, for example, recalled:

> **Stewart:** Having said that, when you are shocked, it's not the same result for everybody. As I said earlier, I get the [makes a small reaction] and it's like muscle jump.
>
> **Gill:** Yeah, yeah.
>
> **Stewart:** Some people have to be physically held on the bed. Erm, you talk to people who have been actually physically shocked when they're out and about. I mean like ...
>
> **Stewart's wife:** When it's working.
>
> **Stewart:** ... when it's working. And some people go from the bottom end of the scale really, really, you know, a bit unpleasant, to other guys [laughs] who says it's like being hit by a baseball bat. [Laughter]

Stewart was unaware of being shocked until his ICD underwent a routine check at the pacemaker clinic. He recalled: 'they actually have me down there which is what I went into three weeks ago and then that's when they suddenly turn around and said, "oh it's gone off".' Whether or not this was a full shock or a series of small cardioverting ones is difficult to assess. Interestingly the opposite event can occur when an individual reports their ICD has gone off, but this is not shown on the ICD records (as discussed in the last chapter). This is a recognised phenomenon known as 'phantom shocks' (Juan and Pollack, 2010). It is an incident that is more often likely to occur at night time, as was the case in Timothy's experience:

> **Timothy:** A phantom shock, in my bed, then home in my bed I had two at least, only when I got to [hospital] I hadn't, it wasn't registered, but up here I had two hits. I thought. Whether I was sleeping and dreamt it I don't know, but I definitely had two shocks in my bed, phoned Anne again, she phoned the ambulance, the ambulance came and by this time I was ...
>
> **Gill:** You still had the physical, the tremors and everything afterwards?
>
> **Timothy:** Yes. But, when they read it, it registered nothing.

Inappropriate firing

So in some cases the ICD had fired and the everyday cyborg had not been aware of it, whereas in others, the everyday cyborg experienced the ICD firing when it had not apparently done so. Additionally, a couple of the everyday cyborgs reported receiving what they felt were inappropriate shocks. Inappropriate shocks were identified by two of the everyday cyborgs David and Shawn. Shawn shared how his first shock had been due to the wires being 'overly-sensitive'. This was related, he felt, to the threshold for the shocks being set by the electrophysiologist at implantation as too low:

> **David:** I, you know, if I'm in a cinema, I want to see a film and, er, people, er, quite near just pissing about and talking a lot and if they're nearby you should go over and tell them to shut up, but they were quite far away, so I came out of the film with my friend, and I went up to them afterwards and started ... started an argument with them about making a noise in the cinema. And I was really, really angry and stressed out and as I, kind of, walked away, my device fired. And, you know, I can understand ... you know, I was really agitated and, you know, my heart was hammering ... but, um, I felt strongly that, um ... that one should be able to get into those situations in life and not worry that you're going to have an ...

Gill: Yeah.

David: … electric shot to the heart. So … but the doctor said that my heart was extremely fast and dangerously fast and that's why …

Gill: Uh-huh.

David: … it fired. And they altered the settings a bit after that.

Gill: Did they?

David: Yeah.

Gill: As in the sense that the level of …

David: They made the thresholds, um, higher, I guess, um, so that wouldn't happen again.

However, as I turn to next, shocks were less likely to be explained by device over-sensing but more likely to be explained by the activity of the everyday cyborg.

Something else is in control

Everyday cyborgs explained why the ICD had fired with nearly all linking the event to an activity they had undertaken. Excesses of worry, exercise, alcohol, coffee, excitement or feeling under the weather were identified as ways of explaining why the ICD had discharged a shock and therefore was inserting an element of control by the everyday cyborg. John suggested to me that his shocks were related to do-it-yourself exertions; Cathy suggested that over-exertion and 'something not quite right with the device contributed to her ICD firing'. Timothy had been shocked on two occasions: once in the excitement of a bowling match and on a later occasion when sitting on the couch. Timothy explained that the latter shock was due to his tendency to worry:

> Timothy: I've said about I'm a worrier, so maybe that has got something to do with it … Even now, that last time, beginning of last year, that was when I had one or two incidents … there was worry then, there was a bit of panic then even when the incident happened, shaking and a right, they [clinicians] said a kind of panic attack, as well as something happening and that didn't help it any. I had to try and, Anne's [daughter] told me all this patter with deep breathing, it's easy to say but when this is happening to you.

In some ways, 'blaming' lifestyles is the everyday cyborg's way of taking back control of their body. As David described how he was 'freaked' out when he first received his ICD: 'Well, I mean, it's the … it's just … I guess it's the whole … it's the whole, this is all wrapped up, you know, feelings of control and feelings that something else has control of the core of you, I guess, you know.' As Jackson says, such strategies make us 'authors of meaning rather than victims of circumstance' (Jackson, 2002). In some ways, this finding can be interpreted as a means in which the everyday cyborg attempts to regain control. Or, at least, post-rationalise what had happened. In my informal discussions with cardiologists, they have suggested that within reason, there is little or no relationship between what could be termed the ordinary activity of the everyday cyborg and the ICD discharging shocks.

Permanent removal, semi-removals and temporarily switching off

The ICD can be switched off and deactivated while in the body through placing a magnet over the site of the ICD that will temporarily disable it from sensing and delivering any shocks. This magnetic device can be used to temporarily 'close the eyes of the ICD', as one cardiac electrophysiologist told me. This is done when the everyday cyborg undergoes medical interventions such as an MRI or radiotherapy. This was the case with Alfred, for example, when receiving treatment for his oesophageal cancer. The actual physical removal and replacement of the battery and the generator from the chest cavity itself is done every eight or so years depending on the amount of ICD activity in terms of pacing, cardioversion and shocks. Because David's ICD had only discharged a shock once and, as discussed above, he questioned whether it was appropriate, he had had discussions with his cardiologist about its removal. David, who was one of the 'oldest' cyborgs having received an ICD almost 20 years previously that was implanted into his stomach due to the size of the ICD at that time, discussed how the wires would be left should it ever be removed:

> David: I mean, the … the one I had in before, as I say, er, they … they found it quite difficult to fit into my body, it was quite …

it was so big. Um, but the other thing is that I think when they took it out, I have a feeling that they weren't taking the wires out, um, because they'd been in there for so long and, er, the way that I remember the surgeon talking about it a few years ago ... er, the effect of stripping the wires from my ...

Gill: Yeah.

David: ... veins would be, er ... would be pretty traumatic and, um ...

Gill: Yeah.

David: ... so, you know, if it did ... if it ... if it was removed and wasn't replaced [the ICD], then I'd still have the, kind of, vestiges of it in my body still, um, I guess.

Norman's ICD was placed on the right-hand side of his chest and not the left due to his veins being blocked with infection.[3] Norman's account of his infection highlights how important the wires are to the discharges of the shocks. Two cables with electrodes at the ends are worked through a vein, into the patient's heart, where they transmit electrical signals back to the ICD. As I suggested earlier, the wires can cause the surgeon significant problems entering them correctly into the heart, but once they are in, it is very difficult to remove the wires. Norman spoke about the infection that his ICD caused and the trouble getting the wires back out:

> **Norman:** It took, it took, it was about ten days from having it, having it replaced, so-called, or put back in and the thing going into terrible infection. So, what they had to then do is to take it all out, everything out.
>
> **Gill:** How did you feel about that?
>
> **Norman:** Well it wasn't very nice, because they couldn't get the wire out. And they had to get the wire out from going through my groin to get it into the heart and pull the wire out that way, 'cause they couldn't get it out any other way.

Removing the wires is a procedure generally avoided because of the possibility of clots being formed and breaking free or as Neil said earlier, when drawing the analogy between his body and a ship, because of the 'gunk'.

None of the everyday cyborgs I spoke with had had the ICD removed despite some requesting it. If a cyborg is created by placing a cybernetic system into an organism, then it would seem plausible to suggest the cyborg identity is reversible when the cybernetic system is removed. It is taking the *cyb*ernetic out of the *org*anism. There are pressing ethical questions about the ICD's removal during the dying process. It is the case that because of the ICD the everyday cyborg will not die from an SCA; however, the ICD can continue to shock the heart during the dying process when the heart ceases to function. Gaining consent to switch it off is important, therefore, as is making the everyday cyborg aware that this distressing situation may arise. I talked about this with only a few of the everyday cyborgs relying mostly on them to bring it up in conversation or at times when I could be confident it would not upset anyone present. This was not often, but had occurred in my interview with Graeme who had recalled a mostly benign experience of cyborgisation during which we discussed ownership of the ICD and then removal:

> **Graeme:** Yeah, erm, I suppose [pause] … I suppose … it might be sensible at some stage, erm, to know who, erm, owns and controls the machine.
> **Gill:** I guess. I guess so. I don't know.
> **Graeme:** And … and whether one does have, erm … erm, the … the authority to say to one's specialist, I want this thing either removed or … or switched off.
> **Gill:** In certain circumstances.
> **Graeme:** Yes.

For Cathy, the ICD removal during the dying process was important for other family members. She thought it would be 'shocking', in this case, for her husband:

> I don't know. For me it wouldn't matter to me because I won't be aware of it but potentially for people round about me that could be very alarming and distressing. I'm just thinking from Roger's point of view if he was with me, given how he feels. Even anybody that wasn't connected to me or didn't even know me if it happened in the street or whatever, I think that it would be shocking for them.

Anne, Timothy's daughter, spontaneously mentioned removing the ICD when I met with her and her husband Tom, during an interview about her father Timothy, who was not present:

> **Anne:** Do you know what worries me and I've never thought about it, right, I don't know whether I saw this on 'Casualty'

[a long-running UK drama series set in a hospital] one day, right, but I don't know if I want this to be on the thingy, right, but how does he [Timothy] die?

Gill: Yeah. That's a question, isn't it?

Anne: And I don't know if he's ever thought about that. I don't know if he's ever … well how does he die? The thing goes off to start your heart. In fact, who was it …

Tom: The brain would die. Does it not? Would it not be starved of the oxygen?

Anne: No, you … it would start … it would just shock you and shock you and shock you and shock you 'til somebody switched it off. Somebody …

Tom: I think we should all get them fitted.

Anne: … told me that. Aye, but there's going to come a point that you don't want to still be … it's … medically …

Tom: They take it then … at that stage, you'd be going in to the hospital and the doctor …

Anne: Yes, but how … what kind of horrendous way …

Tom: … would disconnect that.

Anne: Aye. But how much of a horrendous ordeal is that going to be, 'til you … 'til what? 'Til an ambulance arrives? 'Til they decide that it's shocked you 14 times and they've then got to get you to hospital, because you can't just … I mean, who's going to switch it off? You don't just …

Tom: Well it could be the next frigging morning before they switch it off.

Anne: Exactly. So, it's going to shock you all day … aye.

In the UK, NICE has raised the importance of having such a discussion before implantation of the ICD and 'that careful, explicit and shared decision-making about the appropriate use of these technologies in the context of end-of-life care planning is important' (2014: 40–41). Indeed, in his second interview, John noted such information was available. However, he felt that 'there's a real reluctance of any of the medical staff, I think, to speak to people about the real downside of things, you know', and researchers have suggested similar views to those expressed by him (Russo, 2011). My reluctance to raise the issue during interviews attests to the sensitivities involved. With ICDs, associated vulnerabilities may relate to an alienation to the device being in the body as well as the cyborg being under the control of the ICD as opposed to being in control of it. Acclimatisation to the ICD enables it to be viewed as part of their body and a part of their routine day-to-day life, and it was unclear in the very few conversations with the everyday cyborgs about how they felt about permanent deactivation-ending the techno-organic hybrid life.

Conclusions: the dys-appearance of flesh and machines

To paraphrase Simone de Beauvoir, 'one is not born, but rather becomes an everyday cyborg'. There is a unique liminal depth to the bodily modifications – and breadth to the broader social life changes – caused by reliance on a cybernetic device. I have drawn on accounts of individuals and their significant others to show what it was like to acclimatise to a cybernetic device such as an ICD – to put into words what they felt was going on inside their bodies: in this case, the vulnerabilities caused by alienation from implantation and a reconciliation to possible activation. There is a love-hate relationship between the everyday cyborg and their cybernetic devices. On the one hand it can save their life but on the other it does so by producing a new vulnerability.

For most everyday cyborgs I spoke with, the ICD transitioned from an alien physically forced into their body breaching its integrity, to eventually settle not entirely under but not entirely on the skin. The ICD is out of reach of the everyday cyborg, yet can be felt on the inside, even when resting. The ICD casts a shadow, a silhouette, on the skin's surface and thus it can be felt and seen by the everyday cyborg. Its skin silhouette leaves not only a scar, but an imprint where the integrity of the body has been compromised. Usually, the body is an absent experience to the person in everyday living. Becoming a cyborg causes this taken-for-granted absence of the body to change. This is a second-order absence and is termed 'dys-appearance' (Leder, 1990: 91): in other words, a presence.

The area of the chest where the ICD exists becomes a focal point for the everyday cyborg. For the everyday cyborg, the absent absences of the body and organs are not static states but variable, for example, when the body heals the ICD becomes slowly enmeshed into the body, creating a more comfortable form of techno-organic hybridity. Everyday cyborgs live with a machine inside their bodies that they can feel from the inside out; there was a strong sensation of the ICD being inside the body. For the majority, most of the time the sensation was not dwelt upon and the body is, as Leder (1990) would suggest, an absence in the same way as the rest of the visceral is. Acclimatisation to hybridity occurs when the ICD's body presence becomes an absent absence, and the body returns to an absent state. These are variable processes and are always subject to change. Change can occur when the ICD defibrillates or shocks the cyborg's heart.

Organic versus mechanical

The technology is not organic, it is an alien intrusion and not seen as an actual part of them until, that is, it becomes a part of their 'body' (what they are) as well as a part of their subjectivity and beyond (who they are). The everyday cyborg can reinterpret the technology as transitioning from an alien intrusion to becoming a part of them; a part of their body as well as their life. In the case of device implantation, the transformation is through the device's alienation being recast as human. It is not that the human recipient becomes machine, therefore, but the machine that is humanised. It appeared important that part of the acclimation process was in accepting the hybrid body as the individual's new form of embodiment as a cyborg. While the organism becomes cybernetic, the cybernetic also becomes the organism. When organic hybrids are created through transplantation of non-human animal or human materials, the body and subjectivity is altered in light of the body's modification. Here, human subjectivity is not altered through the modification, as it would be if it were a transplant from an organic source. The ambiguous form of embodiment in the case of techno-organic hybridity such as everyday cyborgs does not mean that the subjectivity is altered due to the materiality that is implanted, but that the cybernetic technology is altered when implanted into the body.

The ICD system becomes enmeshed into the body, but this does not mean that a simultaneous acceptance of the everyday cyborg's subjective 'part of me' will ensue. Enmeshment of the device in the body does not necessarily imply acceptance of the new cyborg subjectivity immediately follows. Almost all everyday cyborgs had experienced loss or change in some aspect of their previous life from their cardiac condition, whether it was their home, economic independence, employment, friends, self-confidence or mobility. The ICD did not and could not change the past, but what its functioning did 'for' them could be seen as a benefit. Becoming a techno-organic hybrid created through placing a cybernetic device in a person is not always straightforward. Acclimatisation to cyborg hybridity was challenging for some and overcoming the alien presence is facilitated by coming to accept it as a positive, allowing the everyday cyborg to live their life anew. In short, the changes to the body allow some to return to the life previously lost by their 'broken heart'.

Reaching the point when it is comfortable in being an everyday cyborg, and is a new state that is the end of the journey that began with the ICD being forced into a body which has little space for it. Acclimatisation, the act of getting used to an 'intruder' and the creation of the new cyborg hybridity, is a fluid and complex process. In some cases, acclimatisation can be uneventful, and the ICD is viewed by the everyday cyborg as a positive and is strongly connected with what it does *for* the individual. This is when the ICD recovers the previous identity of the everyday cyborg which was a subjectivity they had lost with the onset of disease or before the SCA. At such times, then, an ICD is said to be 'part of me' or 'it allows me to be who I am'. Both are powerful statements of acceptance when challenges to the body's integrity are overcome, and the altered subjectivity of the person to cyborg is beneficial.

Autonomy and control

Loved ones and significant others experienced a sense of relief that the ICD is a surveillance system, quite literally life insurance, bringing the emergency hospital room inside the cyborg's body. There are several important features of the ICD's C3I, however, that cause new vulnerabilities for the everyday cyborg. Control emerges as a particularly important dimension by creating vulner-ability in two ways. The first is where the everyday cyborg cannot reach the ICD, resulting in the ICD being out of their physical control. Implantation necessarily causes vulnerability issues because the ICD is implanted and not physically accessible. This is a frustrating paradox in that while the ICD is so close within the cyborg (quite literally inside of them) at the same time, it is outwith their physical control. The second vulnerability results from their lack of control over the device. The ICD's autonomy diminishes the individual's autonomy over it. The ICD can function without a human operator and is capable of self-autonomous actions. The ICD has an element of control in the way that it can cause changes to the heart and its rhythm. The everyday cyborg is under the control of the ICD and is subjected to its actions, whether defined by them or others, as appropriate or not.

Technology often acts in uncertain and unpredictable ways, whether faults in the hardware with wires becoming loose or in the sensing ability of a device to react to what is deemed appropriate in terms of activity or appropriate levels. However, what seemed more disruptive was when the ICD was functioning appropriately and as it was intended to do by shocking the everyday cyborg's heart out of a potentially lethal heart rate. To reconcile the ways that cybernetic control is implemented within the everyday cyborg, the everyday cyborg reasserts their control by narrating how it was their actions that had caused the ICD to discharge. It was common during interviews that a reason was offered as to how the everyday cyborg caused the device to activate whether it was by excessive exercise, consumption or concern. Blaming their actions thus reinserts their control over the autonomy of the device, and is an activity that as human beings we are relatively accomplished at doing:

> Nursing ill-will towards an enemy, cursing an errant computer, kicking a flat tyre, or pitying oneself … will not necessarily effect any change in the behaviour of the object or other, but may reverse one's experience of one's relationship with it. One becomes, imaginatively and retrospectively, the determining subject of the events that reduced on to the status of the object … as actors rather than acted upon, as authors of meaning rather than victims of circumstance.
>
> (Jackson, 2002: 338)

Notes

1 Stewart had an ICD and like most ICDs it has the ability to pace his heart, before then emitting a small series of shocks known as cardioversion, preparing for shock therapy.

2 www2.warwick.ac.uk/fac/med/research/hsri/emergencycare/ prehospitalcare/jrcalcstakeholderwebsite/guidelines/the_implantable_ cardioverter_defibrillator_icd_2006.pdf) (accessed April 2020).

3 He was typical of those that were said to be able to feel their device inside the body: 'Yeah, the device is there, you can feel it … And then I can feel here, there's a wire.' When I asked whether he 'twiddled' with the wire, he responded that he hadn't, although this has been found to be an issue in the medical literature (Nicholson, Tuohy and Tilkemeier, 2003).

Conclusion: Towards a future of techno-organic hybridity

In ending, I revisit the philosophical thought experiment of the 'Ship of Theseus' that was posed in the beginning. A starting point is the question: how much of The Ship can be replaced before it is no longer the same ship? I have explored how much of a human body needs replacing before it is no longer the same body, or indeed the same person. I expanded the philosophical question to include more sociological nuances such as going beyond not only how much requires replacing, but of what? Where in the body do the replacements occur? Are there different types and kinds of materials that could be used to repair and replace the body? To what effects? The technologies of human, animal and mechanical that could be used to restore the body are socially constructed within a nexus of human relationships defining them as human/non-human, male/female, natural/artificial, technological/organic, persons/species and clean/dirty. The way meanings are associated with these materials have consequences for identity and control; of reflexivity and the experiential; of matter and modality; and form and function.

A sociology of embodiment

In researching the lived forms of embodiment through the biomedical practices of organ transplantation, xenotransplantation and cyborgisation, I demonstrate how the experience of embodiment is based on a subjectivity intimately tied to an individual's body. However, there is no paradox in experiencing being a body or having a body as embodiment is ambiguous. I began with following a philosophical path, bringing Descartes' Cartesian Dualism which implies an individual 'has a body' in the same way that they might have a car into conversation with Merleau-Ponty's 'being a body'. Cartesian Dualism is still relevant as modern understandings of what a person is is focused on the brain as the most vital bodily part and that the self is materialised in the brain. Social understandings of self highlight the brain's importance in the experience of cognition, for example. However, I have suggested that the experience of embodiment does not mean that identity is solely located there. Indeed, to put it another way, although I have a brain, I am not a brain.

In contrast, there is a diffuse sense of identity that is bodily located, through, for example, adding my sociological caveats such that unlike Merleau-Ponty's 'embodiment as experience' I have focused upon 'experience as embodiment'. However, Merleau-Ponty's emphasis on the person associating themselves with their body is a key element to bring to the discussion. I have suggested the experience of embodiment is important when an individual's body is modified through transplantation, amputation or cyborgisation. Such body modification creates a body that is no longer absent for the individual; this absence was a taken-for-granted assumption because in our daily lives our bodies have to be part of the background and not at the forefront; otherwise, the continuous focus on our bodies and our relationship to them would hinder and obstruct our day-to-day activities. The body becomes a focal point of experience, creating a reflection that causes the body to be constructed as a separate entity while also being that body. To separate it out, there was unity beforehand. The body through modification of its composition is now an 'absent absence'. This makes the body a presence through the conditions of reflection on having and being a body. I am, and I have, an ambiguity of embodiment. Leder's (1990) 'absent absence' applies as much to the integrity of the body as it does to the image. The integrity of the body's invisible spaces is as important to identity as the visible image. The dermal layer of the body when breached by biomedical practices that insert organs or technology is marked by the entry incision on the surface that allowed the external world in, sometimes by force given how little space there is inside.

Triad of I

The outside-in is the inside-out. The body is one whose identity includes an outside image and an inside integrity and constitutes the Triad of I. Unlike the uncertainty of embodiment, beliefs about human organs are based on a shared understanding that all share the biological condition of humanness. A lived embodied approach to theoretical discussions about embodiment is a recognition of how the reflective dimensions of embodiment are implicated when changes to the interior body are made with organic materials that are similar in terms of species. Recipients know when they receive a human organ. This universality is matched with the knowledge that despite the shared human condition, there is a uniqueness to everyone, and this contributes to the narratives told about the organs, or as Parry calls it, to their 'social life' (Parry, 2018). These socially constructed characteristics of individuality are projected onto the outside body but also the inside of the body. The body is one whose identity includes an outer image and inside integrity. Organ transplants are fleshy. They originate from another body which was human and therefore characteristics such as gender and others such as lifestyle choices can be created about the donor by the recipient. In Chapter 1, the transference of personal characteristics from the donor's organ alters the recipient's sub-jectivity and is a finding that has been reported since the early days of organ transplantation. Female organs are said to be infused with femininity, whereas male organs are associated with ideals of strength.

Moreover, biomedical practices such as organ transplantation and cyborgisation show how embodiment extends beyond an individualised alteration of subjectivity to include living in a social world with others in it. To some extent, what is placed inside the body will affect how the person will relate to others and how they interact in the surrounding space. Body modifications and subject-ivity alterations affect others such as friends and family who are close to the implanted or transplanted techno-hybrid individual. For example, the everyday cyborg is affected by other people and environments that may damage, intentionally or unintentionally, the ICD and, by implication, the everyday cyborg.

It has to be you or me

Partly due to the idea of donor organs being contaminated with their previous identity, replacing a human organ with another human organ brings to the fore reflective social processes by the individual about their experiential aspects of embodiment. When human organs require repair or replacement, the preferred option from human, animal or mechanical will be from human and as similar to the recipient as possible. Repair to the body through regeneration and of 3-D bioprinting maintains the boundaries of the recipient's embodiment from others and negates any risks to subjectivity. These novel findings show the preferred option for repairing the human body is with an organ that came from the same human body (e.g. in the case of 3-D bioprinting), or from a donor who is known or related. In the survey reported in Chapter 2, young adults expressed a firm preference for organs from a known donor. This can be interpreted as an attempt to distance the recipient from possible characteristics from a deceased donor that is a stranger. The danger of an organ from a stranger is a possible subjectivity alteration via contamination but in unknown ways. Actual stories about an anonymous donor given by transplant recipients are consistent with this fear of being contaminated with unknown characteristics. Various explanations have been put forward for the mechanism of this identity transfer including biological (cell memory or as genetic composition); pharmacological (effect of immunosuppressants); and I have emphasised the process of 'contamination' that tells how this happens and incorporates the stories told by recipients (Sanner, 2001a, Sanner, 2001b). It is how donor recipients make the unknown known by creating narratives about a donor they have never met and know very little about.

'Dirty pigs'

If a recipient's subjectivity is altered through contamination from the donor's human fleshy organs, then there is a risk that other fleshy organs might do the same. Non-human animal organs are thought to have the same potential to cause subjectivity alterations to the recipients. Like inter-species contamination between humans, intra-species procedures such as xenotransplantation make it possible to modify the integrity of the recipient's body, altering subjectivity. Chapter 2 (the survey with young people and the focus group research) demonstrates some participants believe human and non-human organic sources, such as from a pig, not only modifies the body but can alter subjectivity. An organ from a pig placed into the human body has the potential to contaminate the body and to make the recipient like the pig (and there are beliefs about 'dirty pigs' for example). Fleshy organic parts, therefore, do have a story of a life previously lived and although there are specific social, cultural and religious beliefs about the consumption of meat and pork, the repugnance wisdom of a 'yuck' reaction to xenotransplantation I have argued, based on the findings from this aspect of the research, is more than prescriptions about vegetarianism and food consumption. Instead, the 'yuck' is related to fundamental questions and perceived threats to the boundaries between humans and other species. Should xenotransplantation and 3-D bioprinting prove successful, Varela suggests:

> We are left to invent a new way of being human where bodily parts go into each other's bodies, redesigning the landscape of boundaries in the habit of what we are so definitively used to call distinct bodies … One day it will be said: I have a pig's heart. Or from stem cells they will graft a new liver or kidney.
>
> (Varela, 2001: 260)

Fleshy organic parts are associated with the identity of those they were once part of.

The current challenge of overcoming biological rejection, which is slowing the progress of xenotransplanting whole animal organs appears to be matched with a cultural one. Using animal parts on a small scale is acceptable and regularly undertaken, such as porcine valves being used as heart valves. Less is enough in these situations. On the one hand, there is a reliance on the biological and physiological similarity between humans and non-human animals for the latter to facilitate therapeutic regimes and medical research.

On the other hand, there is an inherent rejection of shared resemblances when it comes to procedures such as xenotransplantation. This might partly explain why attention is increasingly focusing on the future possibilities of using bio-, nano- and

info-technologies and using genetics, microbes, devices and pharmaceutical interventions, all of which appear to be moving away from
the potentialities that non-human organs might afford. Indeed, part
of this move away from xenotransplantation may be ideologic-
ally based, with the introduction of the term 'non-human animals'
used by animal activists especially, to show that animals demonstrate elements of cognition and emotion. Hence, rights with such
associated (human) personhood should be applied to animals.
Given these countervailing tendencies (an increasing recognition
of the value of non-human animal cellular materiality for human
therapy, while at the same time a greater awareness of the rights of
non-human animals as social beings), there may be a preference for
machines in the flesh.

'Clean machines'

In the survey conducted with young adults reported in Chapter 2,
a mechanical implant was preferred to that of a non-human animal
one. Some recipients were hesitant about a mechanical implant, as
it was perceived as being unnatural and uncomfortable and indeed
a few of the everyday cyborgs echoed this view when sharing their
actual experiences. Preferring not to have a mechanical implant was
related to ideas about reliable functioning, whereby machines break,
rust and malfunction. Quotes such as 'technology and machines
break more often than natural things', and 'it could function wrong
and destroy the inside of my body', are reflective of such a stance.
Indeed, in the later interviews I conducted with everyday cyborgs,
exploring their love-hate relationship with their technology, ICDs
do not represent a threat to subjectivity via contamination in the
manner that a fleshy organ from a human or animal might; however, as reported in the interviews, the ICD does have the potential
to cause infection and to malfunction.

In interviews with everyday cyborgs that I discussed in Chapter 4,
cybernetic modifications to the body do not result in a person being
less human, because less of their body is human. Alteration of what
you are (in the material bodily sense) does not affect who you are
(subjectivity) in the case of creating techno-organic hybrids such
as everyday cyborgs. Simply, a machine has no social history that

is connected to another living being (human/non-human animal, living/dead) in the way that organs have. However, alteration of what you are (in the material bodily sense) does affect who you are (subjectivity) in the case of organ transplantation.

The machine is a different type of material made by a human but never from the body of one. The cybernetic technology is not fleshy and has no previous association with any living being. There is no risk therefore of contamination of characteristics from the source as appears to be the case with fleshy human or animal organs. Technological additions are not assumed to turn the person into a robot as would be the case when altering subjectivity in the way that another human can or non-human animal transplants are assumed to do. Mechanical augmentation has more functional implications for these dimensions of embodiment. Mechanical additions are 'clean' in form but may harness 'potentiality' to save a life and can cause pain by doing so (Helmreich, 2013).

Machines do not have a fleshy origin; they are a different type of materiality unsullied by flesh that can contaminate. The story of devices is one that highlights that machines break, parts wear out and malfunctions are common. Using cybernetics to repair human bodies alters subjectivity in a very different way than organs from human and non-human animals do. The flesh has a story that can cause contamination, whereas the machine is created that can occasionally cause infection. It can malfunction, and inappropriate shocks were said to have been experienced by some. Their implantation does not result in the identity transformations reported by some human organ transplant recipients or envisioned by views about xenotransplantation. The consequences of becoming part cybernetic do not involve any organic additions that are supposed to alter subjectivity as is the case in using a person or a pig. The machine was not previously embodied and cannot contaminate. Nevertheless, the ICD can affect identity in the social world through limiting the patient's ability to socialise, for example. The individual has a unique identity as an everyday cyborg which has nothing in common with the celluloid monster by the technological adaptations that sci-fiction creates and popularises. The only elements that are shared between the sci-fi monster and the everyday cyborg are that they are both more likely to be male.

ICD: cybernetics (cyb) and organisms (org)

However, reliance on biomedical technologies in the form of medical devices to repair organs has been on-going for quite some time, and these technologies are arguably becoming increasingly autonomous, reactive and communicative – the C3I. The application of such smart technologies has the real potential to excite the fears cautioned by Baudrillard insofar as they necessitate the implantation of cybernetic technologies into the human body, masking and hiding what the device (or those hacking into it) might be communicating or interfering with in its commands. What greater ontological insecurity could there be than that created by a device that is in control and autonomous ironically through an intimacy that makes it outwith individual control and out of sight of others. Then cybernetic *technology can give autonomy while simultaneously taking it away.* This loss of control on the part of the everyday cyborg may be key to understanding their vulnerability. Unlike bionics, prosthetics and implantable medical devices, such as CIs and glucose sensors, the ICD functioning is to intervene in a specific and rare instance of an irregular heart rhythm. The everyday cyborg can do nothing either in the case of the cybernetic device functioning or indeed malfunctioning. The ICD causes vulnerability and reflects the lack of autonomy the everyday cyborg has over the ICD that essentially has the control to save his/her life.

If the ICD performs its life-saving function and discharges shocks, the event is explained retrospectively by most everyday cyborgs locating their actions as the reason for the discharge. This reasserts some control over the device (rather than acknowledging the device is in control) and they could therefore blame either themselves through emphasising excesses on their part (worry, exercise, caffeine) or the vulnerabilities in the device (the parameters for shocks are set too low; the leads have broken; the ICD mis-sensed). The everyday cyborg can offer explanations, placing themselves as an agent of the activity and not as a victim of circumstance.

Re-appropriating the term cyborg for our everyday application reinserts issues about what cyborgs need to live happy and fulfilling lives; what kind of support they and their significant others might find useful; as well as what type of information and understanding is required to acclimatise to new techno-organic hybridity. Suppose there is a need to understand and empower those with varying abilities, then a moral and political requirement needs to recognise and celebrate those that are hybrid and materially diverse. There are lessons in what active and meaningful implantation means for the individual. ICDs can cause their cyborgs and their significant others emotional, physiological, psychological and social challenges that are rarely made visible – a cyborg individual or implanted group identification thus reawakens interest in the hybrid condition, leading us to new understandings about the obstacles as well as the benefits that implants pose. There are unique biomedical challenges regarding altered subjectivities, vulnerabilities with known and unknown others and in a loss/gain of human/cybernetic autonomy.

Acclimatisation

Becoming a cyborg in the everyday means that, for some, there is collateral damage; vulnerabilities created, skin cut and changed, body integrity breached; viscera compromised, relationships reformed, subjectivities altered. There are ways additions of new materiality can become part of the body and part of the person. A person can accept an alien part such as that of an implantable medical device or an organ. Jean-Luc Nancy in *L'intrus* relates his experience of receiving a heart transplant. He describes feelings of alienation created by the 'intruder', a deceased donor's heart organ, supposed by Jean-Luc, to be male:

> THE INTRUDER [L'INTRUS] ENTERS BY FORCE, THROUGH SURPRISE OR RUSE, in any case without the right and without having first been admitted … Once he has arrived, if he remains foreign and for as long as he does so – rather than simply 'becoming naturalized' – his coming will not cease; nor will it cease being in some respect an intrusion; that is to say, being without right, familiarity, accustomedness, or habit, the stranger's coming will not cease being a disturbance and perturbation of intimacy.
>
> (Nancy, 2002)

Jean-Luc Nancy discusses in detail his organ transplant, regarding the multiple intruders in his body, ranging from his own heart to the transplant he received, the immunosuppressants created from a rabbit required to stop his body rejecting the transplant, the shingles, to cancer that eventually 'gnaws' at this body. This is not just about one intrusion from outside but a multiplicity of intrusions by the end of his therapy (Geroulanos and Meyers, 2009). The body, as Nancy suggests, 'is thus my self who becomes my own *intrus* – a self that is already profoundly divided and multiple'. 'And yet it is also the "self", the "I" that re-sews at the end' (2002: 15).

Experiencing inorganic/organic hybrid embodiment is a process whereby the transplant or the implant is alien. This alienation is a different experience to the perceptual foreignness of inner organs. The foreignness of our inside organs is a frequent absence that an individual has experienced since birth. However, both transplants and implants leave marks and scars on the body as visible reminders of where breaches into the body's inside and integrity occurred. Both human transplanted organs and implanted technology are unfamiliar alien presences with each either fully or partially disappearing into the familiar foreign space of the interior. There are differences in the depth and reach inside the body. Generally, the ICD may not be submerged to the same extent that a transplanted organ might be. Entry into the body for both, however, is permanently marked by a scar showing where the integrity breach occurred and where a place was found in the viscera for a new alien presence, visually reminding the transplant recipient or everyday cyborg that they are new organic or techno-organic hybrids.

When experience suggests that embodiment is not an event but a process and a journey that is variable in experience and relationship with others, organic transplants and cybernetic implants to the body require varying degrees of acclimatisation to the initial alienation caused by the new artefact. This is because such body modifications recreate bodies that are routinely absent as a presence (or an absent absence). This experience of the body being absent in everyday life is a state where the relationship that a person has with their body is not reflected upon; embodiment is simply forgotten. On the individual level, for the everyday cyborg at least, this is never a status but a journey of change. Their cyborgisation process, in the case of the ICD everyday cyborg, begins after their recovery from a severe illness, disease or a near-death experience. Adjusting to a technological embodiment because of ambiguous intertwinement between body and person can mean that changing a body is not an isolated incident and will have ramifications for identity.

The process of accepting the techno-organic hybrid body becoming 'absent' again in everyday life requires 'acclimatisation'. Acclimatisation is one way of describing the journey of experiencing the body as a presence to an 'absence' once more, in Leder's (1990) terms. Acclimatisation may be relevant for cyborgisation and in organ transplantation too. In her book, *New Organs within Us*, Sanal introduces the Turkish term 'benimseme', referring to 'becoming familiar or feeling at ease with something by making it one's own. It also means internalization ... [and] is a powerful word used to describe how the self, ben, or the ego, can incorporate things' (Sanal, 2011: 4). Varela, when writing about the liver donated to him, reflects on how it did not cause any lasting identity transformation:

> Having the gift in me did not make me become another in any way that experience could attest with any stability. On the contrary, it was the work (again) of temporality that became central: the welcoming, the acceptance of this new form of alterity in spite of immunosuppression, the imaginary elaboration of this intrusion that was willed and wished, regaining the equilibrium from the brutalness of the technology. The images began to disappear, the sudden emotions for the dead giver gave way to a decentring into a larger field of intersubjectivity.
>
> (Varela, 2001: 268)

The images of the deceased donor and the emotions that Varela felt towards them, as well as the donated organ, came to be replaced with a generalised attribution of bonds to others and an awareness of the gift given. This intersubjectivity recognises the connection between individuals that makes the offering of an organ from the deceased possible.

It is for me, not against

Growing comfortable with a hybrid techno-organic status and living with an ICD depends on the everyday cyborg experiencing the ICD as a benefit. Those around them may see the ICD as a benefit because it removes some of the responsibilities of vigilance and oversight they may have had before the cyborgisation process and over the everyday cyborg. Now that the ICD can protect the everyday cyborg from an SCA, family and friends can concentrate on protecting the everyday cyborg from harm caused by their actions. Such protection might be complained about by the everyday cyborg; however, in their accounts, they self-blame and make themselves responsible for the ICD discharging a shock.

The benefit of a hybrid existence through the implantation of a cybernetic device can play a crucial role in shaping how the everyday cyborg acclimatises to their new life. In contrast to the accounts offered by transplant recipients and others, modifying the interior body through transplantation causes subjectivity alterations but the opposite occurs with cyborgisation. The ICD as a cybernetic device is made part of the everyday cyborg – the 'cyb' becomes the 'org'. If a cybernetic device is used, it is not the recipient's subjectivity that is altered, as might be suggested in the case of human or non-human animal transplantation, instead the device becomes a part of the recipient. The ICD becomes both part of the body and the subjectivity of the cyborg.

The everyday cyborg's successful re-acclimatisation to an altered subjectivity of techno-organic hybridity makes their experiences unique when compared to patients who have heart conditions. Living with a device requires adjustments to identity, accepting that the ICD is not an alien and can become part of the person, allowing comfortable co-habiting with cybernetics. Cyborgisation alters materiality and affects subjectivity on one level, creating a need for individuals to undertake the successful acclimatisation process involved in becoming a cyborg. On another level, however, it creates a dependency on the biotechnological fix.

A 21st-century identity crisis

There are factions or groups currently mostly in the US and elsewhere called the 'Transhumanists', who advocate that technoscientific innovations, such as future cybernetic devices, should be embraced because they would make a person 'better' (Savulescu and Bostrom,

2009). 'Better' in this context is used by the Transhumanists to refer to the additional capabilities that other humans do not have (such as the ability to fly). The symbol for the Transhumanist is +H and in their view, the plus sign (+H) represents an addition to the human condition. It demonstrates the possible enhancement of all humanity, despite the normativity of what is and is not 'normal' that arguably underlies much of this type of thinking (Parens, 1998, Baylis and Robert, 2004, Hogle, 2005, Harris, 2007, Buchanan, 2008, Gordijn and Chadwick, 2008, Bostrom and Sandberg, 2009, Savulescu and Bostrom, 2009, Eilers, Grüber and Rehmann-Sutter, 2014). The everyday cyborgs are created through therapeutic modification but not enhanced by their technological modifications (see Daniels, 2000 for a discussion of what the difference is between therapy and enhancement). The speculation in the 1970s regarding the future of the human body and the 'anatomy of the superman' [sic] suggested a basis for enhancing human beings based on the unique qualities of non-human animals:

> The nose of the bloodhound will be ours and the ears of the snake; ours also will be the navigational abilities of certain flying insects, which use vibrating fibers in place of gyros. We will have the adaptions of the sonar of the bat and the porpoise. The eye of the eagle may present problems, since its function must presumably be combined with normal human appearance; yet the bettering man [sic] would have to guess that superman's sight will be better than the eagle at any range.
>
> (Ettinger, 1972: 1)

It appears that current-day discussions regarding enhancing the human body take little recourse of the unique abilities of non-human animal organs – better the 'clean machine' than the 'dirty animal'.

Everyday cyborgs offer a narrative of the contemporary practices of modifying human bodies through bionic, prosthetic and cybernetic technologies that invite a critical understanding of the consequences for the person and whether enhancement does make people better (Van Den Eede, 2015). Increasingly, and running parallel to such a discourse on human enhancement, is a reliance on biomedicine for technological solutions to the developed world health problems. Yet the technoscientific solutions offered in the spheres of biomedicine and enhancement feature mostly male recipients. In so far as we live in a socially structured world, we are subject to the same health and gender inequalities that may become prevalent in a future society of cyborgs that are as entrenched as inequalities are today.

Having raised the spectre of social discrimination in the processes of cyborgisation, it can also be the case that a 21st-century identity crisis is occurring with the boundaries of what is inside-out and outside-in. For cyborg scholar Chris Hables Gray, the process of cyborgisation is akin to that of dying and death as both share a variability but inevitability:

> There are many different types and levels of cyborgization. The incorporated living elements (viral, bacterial, plant, insect, reptile, rodent, avian, mammal), the technological interventions (vaccination, machine prosthesis, genetic engineering, nanobot infection, xenotransplant) and the level of integration (mini, mega, mundane) can all vary, an infinite number of cyborgs, life multiplied by human invention and intervention.
>
> (Gray, 2012: 29)

The identity crisis is created by introducing new vulnerabilities to human beings, being human. The everyday cyborg acclimatises to the fractures that placing an ICD causes in their bodies and lives. Such an ability for individuals to acclimatise to new techno-organic hybridity is a positive, but the downside is that through doing so it masks the presence and magnitude of a 21st-century identity crisis which may explain why it is going on unnoticed. 'They got what they wanted but lost what they had' (Richard Penniman, quoted in Winner, 1993: 371), sums up the often painful ironies of not having any choice. Biomedical nemesis, unlike medical nemesis, centres the ambivalence and vulnerabilities that biomedicine causes as the clinical gaze penetrates the body seeking to implant technoscientific fixes. Biomedical nemesis can be applied to other forms of technoscience interventions that cause unintentional 'un-health' (Illich, 2003). It is a vulnerability that is neither disease nor illness, neither being entirely healthy nor entirely ill, the un-health is euphemistically called the 'new normal' or the 'new different'. The ICD is not only cybernetic through its closed-loop feedback system, with C3I features, but it is the ultimate biomedical nemesis *sine qua non* the iatrogenic device par excellence. The stakes for patient survival have never been so high – without becoming cyborg there is a significant risk of death and yet with it, for some, it can cause vulnerabilities, pain, distress and anxiety – what kind of choice can the individual make when there is no choice to be made at all?

References

Ahmad M., Bloomstein, L., Roelke, M., Bernstein, A. D. and Parsonnet, V. 2000. Patient Attitudes Toward Implanted Defibrillator Shocks. *Pacing and Clinical Electrophysiology*, 23, 934–938.

Allen-Collinson, J. and Hockey, J. 2011. Feeling the Way: Notes Toward a Haptic Phenomenology of Scuba Diving and Distance Running. *International Review for the Sociology of Sport*, 46, 330–345.

Alter, J. 2007. The Once and Future 'Apeman': Chimeras, Human Evolution, and Disciplinary Coherence. *Current Anthropology*, 48, 637–652.

Appel, J. Z., Alwayn, I. P. and Cooper, D. K. 2000. Xenotransplantation: The Challenge to Current Psychosocial Attitudes. *Progress in Transplantation*, 10, 217–225.

Asad, A. L., Anteby, M. and Garip, F. 2014. Who Donates Their Bodies to Science? The Combined Role of Gender and Migration Status among California Whole-body Donors. *Social Science & Medicine*, 106, 53–58.

Ashcroft, F. 2012. *The Spark of Life: Electricity in the Human Body*, London: Penguin Books.

Baudrillard, J. 1996. *The System of Objects*, London and New York: Verso.

Baylis, F. and Robert, J. S. 2004. The Inevitability of Genetic Enhancement Technologies. *Bioethics*, 18, 1–26.

Beck, R. 1987. Possessions and the Extended Self. *Journal of Consumer Research*, 15, 139–163.

Beery, T. A., Sommers, S. M., Hall, J. and King, K. M. 2002. Focused Life Stories of Women with Cardiac Pacemakers. *Western Journal of Nursing Research*, 24, 7–27.

Birke, L. and Michael, M. 1998. The Heart of the Matter: Animal Bodies, Ethics, and Species Boundaries. *Society and Animals*, 6, 245–261.

Birnie, D. H., Sambell, C., Johansen, H., Williams, K., Lemery, R., Green, M. S., Gollob, M. H., Lee, D. S. and Tang, A. S. L. 2007. Use of Implantable Cardioverter Defibrillators in Canadian and US Survivors of Out-of-hospital Cardiac Arrest. *CMAJ*, 177, 41–46.

Bjellanda, I., Dahlb, A. A., Tangen Haugc, T. T. and Neckelmannd, D. 2002. The Validity of the Hospital Anxiety and Depression Scale: An Updated Literature Review. *Journal of Psychosomatic Research*, 52, 69–77.

Bjorn, P. and Markussen, R. 2013. Cyborg Heart: The Affective Apparatus of Bodily Production of ICD Patients. *Science and Technology Studies*, 26, 14–28.

Blackman, L. 2010. Bodily Integrity. *Body & Society*, 16, 1–9.

Blaikie, N. 2007. *Approaches to Social Enquiry*, Cambridge: Polity Press.

Blume, S. S. 1999. Histories of Cochlear Implantation. *Social Science & Medicine*, 49, 1257–1268.

Bona, M. D., Canova, D., Rumiati, R., Russo, F. P., Ermani, M., Ancona, E., Naccarato, R. and Burra, P. 2004. Understanding of and Attitudes to Xenotransplantation: A Survey among Italian University Students. *Xenotransplantation*, 11, 133–140.

Bostrom, N. and Sandberg, A. 2009. Cognitive Enhancement: Methods, Ethics, Regulatory Challenges. *Science and Engineering Ethics*, 15, 311–341.

Bound Alberti, F. 2010. *Matters of the Heart: History, Medicine and Emotion*, Oxford: Oxford University Press.

Brown, N. 1999. Xenotransplantation: Normalizing Disgust. *Science as Culture*, 8, 327–353.

Brown, N. 2009. Beasting the Embryo: The Metrics of Humanness in the Transpecies Embryo Debate. *Biosocieties*, 4, 147–163.

Brown, N. and Michael, M. 2001. Switching between Science and Culture in Transpecies Transplantation. *Science, Technology & Human Values*, 26, 3–22.

Brown, N. and Michael, M. 2004. Risky Creatures: Institutional Species Boundary Change in Biotechnology Regulation. *Health Risk & Society*, 6, 207–222.

Buchanan, A. 2008. Enhancement and the Ethics of Development. *Kennedy Institute of Ethics Journal*, 18, 1–34.

Bunch, T. J., White, R. D., Friedman, P. A., Kottke, T. E., Wu, L. A. and Packer, D. L. 2004. Trends in Treated Ventricular Fibrillation Out-of-hospital Cardiac Arrest: A 17-year Population-based Study. *Heart Rhythm*, 1, 255–259.

Bunch, T. J., White, R. D., Lopez-Jimenez, F. and Thomas, R. J. 2008. Association of Body Weight with Total Mortality and with ICD Shocks among Survivors of Ventricular Fibrillation in Out-of-hospital Cardiac Arrest. *Resuscitation*, 77, 351–355.

Burkitt, I. 1999. *Embodiment, Identity and Modernity*, London: Sage.

Burns J. L., Serber E. R., Keim, S. and Sears, S. F. 2005. Measuring Patient Acceptance of Implantable Cardiac Device Therapy: Initial Psychometric Investigation of the Florida Patient Acceptance Survey. *Journal of Cardiovascular Electrophysiology*, 16, 384–390.

Butler, J. 1993. *Bodies that Matter: On the Discursive Limits of 'Sex'*, London and New York: Routledge.

Buxton, A. E., Lee, K. L., Fisher, J. D., Josephson, M. E., Prystowsky, E. N. and Hafley, G. 1999. A Randomized Study of the Prevention of Sudden Death in Patients with Coronary Artery Disease. *New England Journal of Medicine,* 341, 1882–1890

Buxton, M., Caine, N., Chase, D., Connelly, D., Grace, A., Jackson, C., Parkes, J. and Sharples, L. 2006. A review of the evidence on the effects and costs of implantable cardioverter defibrillator therapy in different patient groups, and modelling of cost-effectiveness and cost–utility for these groups in a UK context. *Health Technology Assessment,* 10, 1–184.

Campbell, C. C., Clark, A. L., Loy, D., Keenan, F. J., Matthews, K., Winograd, T. and Zoloth, L. 2007. The Bodily Incorporation of Mechanical Devices: Ethical and Religious Issues (Part 1). *Cambridge Quarterly of Healthcare Ethics,* 16(2), 229–239.

Canova, D., Bona, M. D., Rumiati, R., Masier, A., Ermani, M., Naccarato, R., Cozzi, E., Ancona, E. and Burra, P. 2006. Understanding of and Attitude to Xenotransplantation among Italian University Students: Impact of a 3-yr University Course. *Xenotransplantation,* 13, 264–271.

Castelnuovo-Tedesco, P. 1973. Organ Transplant, Body Image and Psychosis. *Psychoanalytical Quarterly,* 42, 349–363.

Chakrabarty, A. 2003. Crossing Species Boundaries and Making Human-Nonhuman Hybrids: Moral and Legal Ramifications. *American Journal of Bioethics,* 3, 20–21.

Charmaz, K. 1995. The Body, Identity, and Self: Adapting To Impairment. *Sociological Quarterly,* 36, 4, 657–680.

Chorost, M. 2005. *Rebuilt: How Becoming Part Computer Made Me More Human,* London: Souvenier Press.

Clark, A. 2003. *Natural Born Cyborgs: Minds, Technologies, and the Future of Human Intelligence,* Oxford, Oxford University Press.

Clark, A. 2007. Re-inventing Ourselves: The Plasticity of Embodiment, Sensing, and Mind. *Journal of Medicine and Philosophy,* 32, 263–282.

Clarke, A. E., Mamo, L., Fosket, J. R., Fishman, J. R. and Shim, J. K. 2010. *Biomedicalization: Technoscience, Health, and Illness in the U.S.,* Durham, NC: Duke University Press.

Clynes, M. E. and Kline, N. D. 1960. Cyborgs and Space. *Astronautics,* 5(9), 26–76.

Conesa, C., Ríos, A., Ramírez, P., Sánchez, J., Sánchez, E., Rodríguez, M. M., Martínez, L., Fernández, O. M., Ramos, F., Montoya, M. J. and Parrilla, P. 2006. Attitudes of Primary Care Professionals in Spain Toward Xenotransplantation. *Transplantation Proceedings,* 38, 853–857.

Connell, R. 1995. *Masculinities*, Cambridge: Polity Press.

Cook, J. A., Shah, K. B., Quader, M. A., Cooke, R. H., Kasirajan, V., Rao, K. K., Smallfield, M. C., Tchoukina, I. and Tang, D. G. 2015. The Total Artificial Heart. *Journal of Thoracic Disease*, 7, 2172–2180.

Craig, A. D. 2002. How Do You Feel? Interoception: The Sense of the Physiological Condition of the Body. *Nature Reviews Neuroscience*, 3, 655–666.

Craney, J. M., Mandle, C. L., Munro, B. H. and Rankin, S. 1997. Implantable Cardioverter Defibrillators: Physical and Psychosocial Outcomes. *American Journal of Critical Care*, 6, 445–451.

Crawford, C. S. 2014. *Phantom Limb: Amputation, Embodiment, and Prosthetic Technology*, New York: New York University Press.

Cregan, K. 2006. *The Sociology of the Body: Mapping the Abstraction of Embodiment*, London: Sage.

Crossley, N. 1995. Merleau-Ponty, the Elusive Body and Carnal Sociology. *Body & Society*, 1, 43–63.

Crossley, N. 2001. Embodiment and Social Structure: A Response to Howson and Inglis. *Sociological Review*, 49, 318–326.

Csordas, T. J. (ed.) 1994. *Embodiment and Experience: The Existential Ground of Culture and Self*, Cambridge: Cambridge University Press.

Dalibert, L. 2016. Living with Spinal Cord Stimulation: Doing Embodiment and Incorporation. *Science, Technology, & Human Values*, 41, 635–659.

Daniels, N. 2000. Normal Functioning and the Treatment-Enhancement Distinction. *Cambridge Quarterly of Healthcare Ethics*, 9, 309–322.

Das, V. 2010. Engaging the Life of the Other: Love and Everyday Life. In: M. Lambeck (ed.), *Ordinary Ethics: Anthropology, Language, and Action*, New York: Fordham University Press.

Davie, J. E., Walling, M. R., Ashton Mansour, D. J., Bromham, D., Kishen, M. and Fowler, P. 1996. Impact of Patient Counseling on Acceptance of the Levonorgestrel Implant Contraceptive in the United Kingdom. *Clinical Therapeutics*, 18, 150–159.

Davies, G. 2006. The Sacred and the Profane: Biotechnology, Rationality and Public Debate. *Environment and Planning A*, 38, 423–443.

De Preester, H. and Tsakiris, M. 2009. Body-extension Versus Body-incorporation: Is There a Need for a Body-model? *Phenomenology and the Cognitive Sciences*, 8, 307–319.

Degrazia, D. 2007. Human-animal Chimeras: Human Dignity, Moral Status, and Species Prejudice. *Metaphilosophy*, 38, 309–329.

Dickerson, S. 2002. Redefining Life While Forestalling Death: Living with an Implantable Cardioverter Defibrillator after a Sudden Cardiac Death Experience. *Qualitative Health Research*, 12, 360–371.

Doniger, W. 1995. Transplanting Myths of Organ Transplants. In: S. Younger, R. Fox, and L. O'Connell (eds.), *Organ Transplantation: Meanings and Realities.* Wisconsin: University of Wisconsin Press.

Dougherty, C. M. 1995. Psychological reactions and family adjustment in shock versus no shock groups after implantation of internal cardioverter defibrillator. *Heart and Lung,* 24, 281–291.

Dougherty, C. M. 1997. Family-focused Interventions for Survivors of Sudden Cardiac Arrest. *Journal of Cardiovascular Nursing,* 12, 45–58.

Dougherty, C. M., Pyper, G. P. and Benoliel, J. Q. 2004. Domains of Concern of Intimate Partners of Sudden Cardiac Arrest Survivors after ICD Implantation. *Journal of Cardiovascular Nursing,* 19, 21–31.

Douglas, M. 1966. *Purity and Danger: An Analysis of Pollution and Taboo,* London: Routledge & Kegan Paul.

Douglas, M. 1972. Deciphering a Meal. *Daedalus,* 101, 61–81.

Dunbar, S. B, Kimble, L., Jenkins, L., Hawthorne, M., Dudley, W., Slemmons, M. and Langberg, J. 1999. Association of Mood Disturbance and Arrhythmia Events in Patients after Cardioverter Defibrillator Implantation. *Depression & Anxiety,* 9, 163–168.

Duru, F., Büchi, S., Klaghofer, R., Sensky, T., Buddeberg, C. and Candinas, R. 2001. How Different from Pacemaker Patients Are Recipients of Implantable Cardioverter-defibrillators with Respect to Psychosocial Adaptation, Affective Disorders, and Quality of Life? *Heart,* 85, 375–379.

Eckert, M. and Jones, T. 2002. How Does an Implantable Cardioverter Defibrillator (ICD) Affect the Lives of Patients and Their Families? *International Journal of Nursing Practice,* 8, 152–157.

Eilers, M., Grüber, K. and Rehmann-Sutter, C. 2014. *The Human Enhancement Debate and Disability: New Bodies for a Better Life,* London: Palgrave Macmillan.

Ellenbogen, K. A., Wood, M. A. and Swerdlow, C. D. 2008. The Sprint Fidelis Lead Fracture Story: What Do We Really Know and Where Do We Go from Here? *Heart Rhythm,* 5, 1380–1381.

Emslie, C. and Hunt, K. 2009. Men, Masculinities and Heart Disease: A Systematic Review of the Qualitative Literature. *Current Sociology,* 57, 155–191.

Evans, M. and Lee, E. (eds.) 2002. *Real Bodies: A Sociological Introduction,* New York: Palgrave.

Farr, W., Price, S. and Jewitt, C. 2012. An Introduction to Embodiment and Digital Technology Research: Interdisciplinary Themes and Perspectives. In: *Economic and Social Science Research Council* (ed.), *MODE node,* London: Institute of Education.

Featherstone, M. and Burrows, R. (eds.) 1995. *Cyberspace/Cyberbodies/ Cyberpunk: Cultures of Technological Embodiment,* London: Sage.

Fielding, H. 1999. Depth of Embodiment: Spatial and Temporal Bodies in Foucault and Merleau-Ponty. *Philosophy Today,* 43, 73–85.

Forsberg, A., Bäckman, L. and Möller, A. 2000. Experiencing Liver Transplantation: A Phenomenological Approach. *Journal of Advanced Nursing,* 32, 327–334.

Fovargue, S. 2007. 'Oh Pick Me, Pick Me' – Selecting Participants for Xenotransplant Clinical Trials. *Medical Law Review,* 15(2), 176–219.

Fox, R. and Swazey, J. 1974. *The Courage to Fail: A Social View of Organ Transplants and Dialysis,* Chicago: University of Chicago Press.

Fox, R. C. and Swazey, J. P. 1992. *Spare Parts. Organ Replacement in American Society,* Oxford: Oxford University Press.

Francione, G. 2008. *Animals as Persons: Essay on the Abolition of Animal Exploitation*, Columbia: Columbia University Press.

Francis, J., Johnson, B. and Niehaus, M. 2006. Quality of Life in Patients with Implantable Cardioverter Defibrillators. *Indian Pacing and Electrophysiology Journal,* 6, 173–181.

Freeman, M. and Abou Jaoude, P. 2007. Justifying Surgery's Last Taboo: The Ethics of Face Transplants. *Journal of Medical Ethics,* 33, 76–81.

Friedewald, M. R., Lindner, R. and Wright, D. (eds.) 2006. *Policy Options to Counteract Threats and Vulnerabilities in Ambient Intelligence, SWAMI Deliverable D3: A report to the SWAMI consortium to the European Commission under contract 006507,* http://swami.jrc.es.

Fulton, J., Fulton, R. and Simmons, R. 1987. The Cadaver Donor and the Gift of Life. In: R. Simmons, S. K. Klein, and R. Simmons (eds.), *Gift of Life: The Effects of Organ Donation on Individual, Family and Social Dynamics,* Oxford: Transaction Books.

Gadow, S. 1980. Body and Self: A Dialectic. *Journal of Medicine and Philosophy,* 5, 172–185.

Gardner, J. 2013. A History of Deep Brain Stimulation: Technological Innovation and the Role of Clinical Assessment Tools. *Social Studies of Science,* 43, 707–728.

Gardner, J., Higham, R., Faulkner, A. and Webster, A. 2017. Promissory Identities: Sociotechnical Representations & Innovation in Regenerative Medicine. *Social Science & Medicine,* 174, 70–78.

Gardner, J. and Warren, N. 2019. Learning from Deep Brain Stimulation: The Fallacy of Techno-solutionism and the Need for 'Regimes of Care'. *Medicine, Health Care and Philosophy,* 22, 364–337.

Gardner, J., Warren, N., Addison, C. and Samuel, G. 2019. Persuasive Bodies: Testimonies of Deep Brain Stimulation and Parkinson's on YouTube. *Social Science & Medicine,* 222, 44–51.

Geroulanos, S. and Meyers, T. 2009. A Graft, Physiological and Philosophical: Jean-Luc Nancy's L'intrus. *Parallax,* 15, 83–96.

Gilbert, F. 2017. Deep Brain Stimulation: Inducing Self-Estrangement. *Neuroethics,* 5(6), 1–9.

Glannon, W. 2009. Our Brains Are Not Us. *Bioethics,* 23, 321–329.

Gordijn, B. and Chadwick, R. (eds.) 2008. *Medical Enhancement and Posthumanity,* The Netherlands: Springer.

Gray, C. H. 1995a. *The Cyborg Handbook,* London and New York: Routledge.

Gray, C. H. (ed.) 1995b. *An Interview with Manfred Clynes.* In: C. H. Gray, 1995a. *The Cyborg Handbook,* London and New York: Routledge.

Gray, C. H. 2000. Man Plus: Enhanced Cyborgs and the Construction of the Future Masculine. *Science as Culture,* 9, 277–299.

Gray, C. H. 2001. *Cyborg Citizen: Politics in the Posthuman Age,* New York and London: Routledge.

Gray, C. H. 2011. Homo Cyborg: Fifty Years Old. *Revista Teknokultura,* 8, 83–104.

Gray, C. H. 2012. Cyborging the Posthuman: Participatory Evolution. In: K. Lippert-Rasmussen, M. Rosendahl Thomsen and J. Wamberg (eds.), *The Posthuman Condition: Ethics, Aesthetics and Politics of Biotechnical Challenges.* Aarrhus: Aarrhus University Press.

Gray, R. F., Ray, J., Baguley, D. M., Vanat, Z., Begg, J. and Phelps, P. D. 1998. Cochlear Implant Failure Due to Unexpected Absence of the Eighth Nerve: A Cautionary Tale. *The Journal of Laryngology & Otology,* 112, 646–649.

Green, W. A. and Moss, A. J. 1969. Psychosocial Factors in the Adjustment of Patients with Automatic Implantable Cardiac Pacemakers. *Annual Internal Medicine,* 70, 897–902.

Grosz, E. 1994. *Volatile Bodies: Towards a Corporeal Feminism,* Bloomington: Indiana University Press.

Hacking, I. 2007. Our Neo-Cartesian Bodies in Parts. *Critical Inquiry,* 34, 78–105.

Haddow, G. 2005. The Phenomenology of Death, Embodiment and Organ Transplantation. *Sociology of Health & Illness,* 27, 92–113.

Haddow, G., Bruce, A., Calvert, J., Harmon, S. and Marsden, W. 2010. Not 'Human' Enough to be Human But Not 'Animal' Enough to Be Animal: The Case of the HFEA, Cybrids and Xenotransplantation. *New Genetics and Society,* 29, 3–17.

Haddow, G., Harmon, S. E. and Gilman, L. 2016. Implantable Smart Technologies (IST): Defining the 'Sting' in Data and Device. *Health Care Analysis,* 24(3), 210–227.

Haddow, G., King, E., Kunkler, I. and Mclaren, D. 2015. Cyborgs in the Everyday: Masculinity and Biosensing Prostate Cancer. *Science as Culture,* 24, 484–506.

Halacy, D. S. 1965. *Cyborg: Evolution of the Superman,* New York and Evanston: Harper and Row.

Halperin, D., Heydit-Benjamin, T., Fu, K., Kohno, T. and Maisel, W. 2008a. Security and Privacy for Implantable Medical Devices. *IEEE Pervasive Comput Special Issue Implant Electron,* 7, 30–39.

Halperin, D., Heydt-Benjamin, T. S., Ransford, B., Clark, S. S., Defend, B., Morgan, W. and Fu, K. 2008b. Pacemakers and Implantable Cardiac Defibrillators; Software Radio Attacks and Zero-power Defenses. *Proceedings of the 2008 IEEE Symposium on Security and Privacy,* CA: IEEE Computer Society, 129–142.

Hammill, S. C., Kremers, M. S., Stevenson, L. W., Heidenreich, P. A., Lang, C. M., Curtis, J. P., Wang, Y., Berul, C. I., Kadish, A. H., Al-Khatib, S. M., Pina, I. L., Walsh, M. N., Mirro, M. J., Lindsay, B. D., Reynolds, M. R., Pontzer, K., Blum, L., Masoudi, F., Rumsfeld, J. and Brindis, R. G. 2010. Review of the Registry's Fourth Year, Incorporating Lead Data and Pediatric ICD Procedures, and Use as a National Performance Measure. *Heart Rhythm,* 7, 1340–1345.

Haraway, D. 1991. A Cyborg Manifesto: Science, Technology, and Socialist-Feminism in the Late Twentieth Century. *Simians, Cyborgs and Women: The Reinvention of Nature,* New York: Routledge.

Haraway, D. 2003. *The Companion Species Manifesto: Dogs, People, and Significant Otherness,* Chicago: Prickly Paradigm Press.

Harmon, S., Haddow, G. and Gilman, L. 2015. New Risks Inadequately Managed: The Case of Smart Implants and Medical Device Regulation. *Law, Innovation and Technology,* 7, 231–252.

Harris, J. 2005. Sparrows, Hedgehogs and Castrati: Reflections on Gender and Enhancement. *Journal of Medical Ethics,* 37, 262–266.

Harris, J. 2007. *Enhancing Evolution: The Ethical Case for Making Better People,* Princeton: Princeton University Press.

Harrison, P. 2000. Making Sense: Embodiment and Sensibilities of the Everyday. *Environment and Planning D: Society and Space,* 18, 497–517.

Hayles, K. 1995. The Life Cycle of Cyborgs: Writing the Posthuman. In: C. H. Gray, H. J. Figueroa-Sarriera and S. Mentor (eds.), *The Cyborg Handbook,* New York and London: Routledge.

Hegel, M. T., Griegel, L. E., Black, C., Goulden, L. and Ozahowski, T. 1997. Anxiety and Depression in Patients Receiving Implanted Cardioverter-defibrillators: A Longitudinal Investigation. *International Journal of Psychiatry in Medicine,* 27, 57–69.

Helman, C. 1991. *Body Myths,* London: Chatto and Windus.

Helmreich, S. 2011. What was Life? Answers from Three Limit Biologies. *Critical Inquiry,* 47, 671–696.

Henwood, F., Kennedy, H. and Miller, N. (eds.) 2001. *Cyborg Lives: Women's Technobiographies*, York: Raw Nerve Books.

Hogle, L. F. 2005. Enhancement Technologies and the Body. *Annual Review of Anthropology*, 34, 695–716.

House, L. M., Mckay, R. E., Eagan, J. T. and Mccormick, Z. L. 2018. Nocturnal Phantom Shock Cessation with Zolpidem. *Heart & Lung*, 47, 76–79.

Howson, A. 2004. *The Body in Society: An Introduction*, Cambridge, Polity Press.

Howson, A. and Inglis, D. 2001. The Body in Sociology: Tensions Inside and Outside Sociological Thought. *Sociological Review*, 49, 297–317.

Høystad, M. O. 2007. *A History of the Heart*, London: Reaktion Books.

Idvall, M. 2006. The Xenotransplantation Narratives of Nine Type 1 Diabetic Patients with Renal Failure. *Xenotransplantation*, 13, 509–511.

Ihde, D. 1990. *Technology and the Lifeworld: From Garden to Earth*, Bloomington: Indiana University Press.

Illich, I. 2003. Medical Nemesis. *Journal of Epidemiology and Community, Health*, 57, 919–922.

Inglis, D. and Howson, A. 2002. Sociology's Sense of Self: A Response to Crossley and Shilling. *Sociological Review*, 50, 136–139.

Insurers., A. O. B. 2004. Genetic Testing and Insurance: ABI Code of Practice on Genetic Testing. Compliance Report and Data Analysis for 2002.

Irvine, J., Dorian, P. and Baker, B. 2002. Quality of Life in the Canadian Implantable Defibrillator Study. *American Heart Journal*, 144, 282–289.

Jackson, M. 2002. Familiar and Foreign Bodies: A Phenomenological Exploration of the Human-Technology Interface. *Journal of the Royal Anthropological Institute*, 8, 333–346.

Jenkins, N. 2013. Dementia and the Inter-embodied Self. *Social Theory and Health*, 12(2), 1–13.

Juan, E. A. and Pollack, M. 2010. Phantom Shocks in Patients with an Implantable Cardioverter Defibrillator. *Journal of Emergency Medicine*, 38, 22–24.

Kass, L. 1985. Thinking about the Body. *Hastings Center Report*, 15(1), 20–30.

Kass, L. 2002. *Life, Liberty and the Defense of Dignity: The Challenge for Bioethics*, San Francisco: Encounter Books.

Kelley, A. S., Mehta, S. S. and Reid, M. C. 2008. Management of Patients with ICDs at the End Of Life (EOL): A Qualitative Study. *American Journal of Hospice & Palliative Care*, 25, 440–446.

Kirkup, G., Janes, L., Woodward, K. and Hovenden, F. 1999. *The Gendered Cyborg: A Reader*, London and New York: Routledge.

Klaming, L. and Haselager, P. 2013. Did My Brain Implant Make Me Do It? Questions Raised by DBS Regarding Psychological Continuity, Responsibility for Action and Mental Competence. *Neuroethics, 6,* 527–539.

Knoppers, B. M. and Joly, Y. 2007. Our social genome? *Trends in Biotechnology,* 25(7), 824–828.

Kraemer, F. 2013. Authenticity or Autonomy? When Deep Brain Stimulation Causes a Dilemma. *Journal of Medical Ethics, 39,* 757–760.

Kranenburg, L. W., Kerssens, C., Ijzermans, J. N., Zuidema, W., Weimar, W. and Busschbach, J. J. 2005. Reluctant Acceptance of Xenotransplantation in Kidney Patients on the Waiting List for Transplantation. *Social Science and Medicine,* 61, 1828–1834.

Kuhl, E. A., Dixit, N. K., Walker, R. L., Conti, J. B. and Sears, S. F. 2006. Measurement of Patient Fears About Implantable Cardioverter Defibrillator Shock: An Initial Evaluation of the Florida Shock Anxiety Scale. *Pacing and Clinical Electrophysiology,* 29, 614–618.

Kushner, T. and Belliotti, S. 1985. Baby Fae: A Beastly Business. *Journal of Medical Ethics,* 11, 187–183.

Lampert, R., Joska, T., Burg, M., Batsford, W., Mcpherson, C. and Jain, D. 2002. Emotional and Physical Precipants of Ventricular Arrhythmia. *Circulation,* 106, 1800–1805.

Le Breton, D. 2015. From Disfigurement to Facial Transplant: Identity Insights. *Body & Society,* 21, 3–23.

Leder, D. 1990. *The Absent Body,* Chicago: University of Chicago Press.

Levine, G. N., Steinke, E. E., Bakaeen, F. G., Bozkurt, B., Cheitlin, M. D., Conti, J. B., Foster, E., Jaarsma, T., Kloner, R. A., Lange, R. A., Lindau, S. T., Maron, B. J., Moser, D. K., Ohman, E. M., Seftel, A. D. and Stewart, W. J. 2012. Sexual Activity and Cardiovascular Disease: A Scientific Statement from the American Heart Association. *Circulation,* 125(9), 1058–1072.

Lipscomb, K. J., Linker, N. J. and Fitzpatrick, A. P. 1998. Subpectoral Implantation of a Cardioverter Defibrillator Under Local Anaesthesia. *Heart,* 79, 253–255.

Lipsman, N. I. R. and Glannon, W. 2012. Brain, Mind and Machine: What Are the Implications of Deep Brain Stimulation for Perceptions of Personal Identity, Agency and Free Will? *Bioethics,* 27(9), 465–470. doi: 10.1111/j.1467-8519.2012.01978.x. Epub 2012 Jun 10. PMID: 22681593.

Lock, M. 1995a. Contesting the Natural in Japan: Moral Dilemmas and Technologies of Dying. *Culture, Medicine and Psychiatry,* 19, 1–38.

Lock, M. 1995b. Transcending Mortality: Organ Transplants and the Practice of Contradictions. *Medical Anthropology Quarterly, 9,* 390–398.

Luderitz, B., Jung, W., Deister, A., Marneros, M. and Manz, M. 1994. Patient Acceptance of Implantable Cardioverter Defibrillator Devices: Changing Attitudes. *American Heart Journal,* 127, 1179–1184.

Lundin, S. 1999. The Boundless Body: Cultural Perspectives on Xenotransplantation. *Ethnos,* 64, 5–31.

Lundin, S. 2002. Creating Identity with Biotechnology: The Xenotransplanted Body as the Norm. *Public Understanding of Science,* 11, 333–345.

Lundin, S. and Idvall, M. 2003. Attitudes of Swedes to Marginal Donors and Xenotransplantation. *Journal of Medical Ethics,* 29, 186–192.

Lundin, S. and Widner, H. 2000. Attitudes to Xenotransplantation: Interviews with Patients Suffering from Parkinson's Disease Focusing on the Conception of Risk. *Transplantation Proceedings,* 32, 1175–1176.

Lupton, D. 2013. Infant Embodiment and Interembodiment: A Review of Sociocultural Perspectives. *Childhood,* 20, 37–50.

MacKellar, C., and Jones, D. A. 2012. *Chimera's Children: Philosophical and Religious Perspectives on Human-NonHuman Experimentation,* London: Continuum Books.

Madison, G. B. 1981. *The Phenomenology of Merleau-Ponty: A Search for the Limits of Consciousness,* Ohio: Ohio University Press.

Magyar-Russell, G., Thombs, B. D., Cai, J. X., Baveja, T., Kuhl, E. A., Singh, P. P., Barroso, M. M. B., Arthurs, E., Roseman, M., Amin, N., Marine, J. E. and Ziegelstein, R. C. 2011. The Prevalence of Anxiety and Depression in Adults with Implantable Cardioverter Defibrillators: A Systematic Review. *Journal of Psychosomatic Research,* 71, 223–231.

Maisel, W. H., Sweeney, M. O., Stevenson, W. G., Ellison, K. E. and Epstein, L. M. 2001. Recalls and Safety Alerts Involving Pacemakers and Implantable Cardioverter-Defibrillators. *Journal of American Medical Association,* 286, 793–799.

Manning Stevens, S. 1997. Sacred Heart and Secular Brain. In: D. Hillman and C. Mazzio (eds.), *The Body in Parts: Fantasies of Corporeality in Early Modern Europe.* London and New York: Routledge.

Marshall, P., Ketchell, A. and Maclean, J. 2011. Comparison of Male and Female Psychological Outcomes Related to Implantable Cardioverter Defibrillators (COMFORTID). *European Journal of Cardiovascular Nursing,* 11, 313–321.

Martindale, A.-M. and Fisher, P. 2019. Disrupted Faces, Disrupted Identities? Embodiment, Life Stories and Acquired Facial 'Disfigurement'. *Sociology of Health & Illness,* 41(8), 1503–1509.

Martinez-Alarcon, L., Rios, A., Conesa, C., Alcaraz, J., Gonzalez, M. J., MONTOYA, M., Fernandez, O. M., Majado, M., Ramirez, P. and Parrilla, P. 2005. Attitude Toward Xenotransplantation in Kidney and Liver Patients on the Transplant Waiting List. *Transplantation Proceedings,* 37, 4107–4110.

Mentor, S. 2011. The Coming of the Mundane Cyborg. *Revista Teknokultura*, 8, 47–61.

Merleau-Ponty, M. 2012 (1945). *Phenomenology of Perception*, London and New York: Routledge.

Mironov, V., Kasyanov, V. and Markwald, R. R. 2011. Organ Printing: From Bioprinter to Organ Biofabrication Line. *Current Opinion in Biotechnology*, 22, 667–673.

Mohiuddin, M. M., Singh, A. K., Corcoran, P. C., Thomas III, M. L., Clark, T., Lewis, B. G., Hoyt, R. F., Eckhaus, M., Pierson III, R. N., Belli, A. J., Wolf, E., Klymiuk, N., Phelps, C., Reimann, K. A., Ayares, D. and Horvath, K. A. 2016. Chimeric 2C10R4 anti-CD40 Antibody Therapy is Critical for Long-term Survival of GTKO.hCD46.hTBM Pig-to-primate Cardiac Xenograft. *Nature Communications*, 7, 11138.

More, M. and Vita-More, N. (eds.) 2013. *The Transhumanist Reader: Classical and Contemporary Essays on the Science, Technology, and Philosophy of the Human Future*, London: Wiley-Blackwell.

Murray, C. D. 2004. An Interpretative Phenomenological Analysis of the Embodiment of Artificial Limbs. *Disability and Rehabilitation*, 26, 963–973.

Nancy, J. L. 2002 L'Intrus. *The New Centennial Review*, 2, 1–14.

Nathoo, A. 2007. The Transplanted Heart: Surgery in the 1960s. In: J. Peto (ed.), *The Heart*. New Haven and London: Yale University Press.

Newman, H. D. and Carpenter, L. M. 2013. Embodiment without Bodies? Analysis of Embodiment in US-based Pro-breastfeeding and Anti-male Circumcision Movements. *Sociology of Health & Illness*, 36(5), 639–654.

NICE. 2014. Implantable Cardioverter Defibrillators for Arrythmias: Review of Technology Appraisal 11. www.nice.org.uk/guidance/ta314 (accessed January 2015).

Nicholson, W. J., Tuohy, K. A. and Tilkemeier, P. 2003. Twiddler's Syndrome. *New England Journal of Medicine*, 348, 1726–1727.

North Sound London Cardiac Arrythmia Network. 2013. Guidelines for deactivating implantable cardioverter defibrillators (ICDs) in people nearing the end of their life (accessed April 2014).

O'Gara, P. T., Kushner, F. G., Ascheim, D. D., Casey, D. E., Chung, M. K., De Lemos, J. A., Ettinger, S. M., Fang, J. C., Fesmire, F. M., Franklin, B. A., Granger, C. B., Krumholz, H. M., Linderbaum, J. A., Morrow, D. A., Newby, L. K., Ornato, J. P., Ou, N., Radford, M. J., Tamis-Holland, J. E., Tommaso, C. L., Tracy, C. M., Woo, Y. J. and Zhao, D. X. 2013. 2013 ACCF/AHA Guideline for the Management of ST-Elevation Myocardial Infarction: Executive Summary: A Report of the American College of Cardiology Foundation/American Heart Association Task Force on Practice Guidelines. *Journal of the American College of Cardiology*, 61, 485–510.

Oetler, M. 1995. From Captain America to Wolverine: Cyborgs in Comic Books, Alternative Images of Cybernetic Heroes and Villians. In: C. Gray, H. Figueroa-Sarriera and S. Mentor (eds.), *The Cyborg Handbook*, New York: Routledge.

Office of National Statistics. 2018. Leading Causes of Death in the UK. www.ons.gov.uk/peoplepopulationandcommunity/healthandsocialcare/causesofdeath/articles/leadingcausesofdeathuk/2001to2018#uk-leading-causes-of-death-for-all-ages (accessed February 2021).

Oudshoorn, N. 2015. Sustaining Cyborgs: Sensing and Tuning Agencies of Pacemakers and Implantable Cardioverter Defibrillators. *Social Studies of Science,* 45, 56–76.

Oudshoorn, N. 2016. The Vulnerability of Cyborgs: The Case of ICD Shocks. *Science, Technology & Human Values,* 40, 3, 338–367.

Ozawa-De Silva, C. 2002. Beyond the Body/Mind? Japanese Contemporary Thinkers on Alternative Sociologies of the Body. *Body and Society,* 8, 21–38.

Palacios-Cena, D., Losa-Iglesias, M. E., Salvadores-Fuentes, P., Alonso-Blanco, C. and Fernandez-de-las-Penas, C. 2011. Experience of Elderly Spanish Men with an Implantable Cardioverter-defibrillator. *Geriatrics & Gerontology International,* 11, 320–327.

Parens, E. 1998. Is Better Always Good? The Enhancement Project. *Hastings Center Report,* 28, U1-S17.

Parry, B. 2018. The Social Life of 'Scaffolds': Examining Human Rights in Regenerative Medicine. *Science, Technology, & Human Values,* 43, 95–120.

Pearsall, P. 1999. *The Heart's Code: Tapping the Wisdom and Power of Our Heart Energy (the New Findings about cellular memories and Their Role in the Mind/Body/Spirit Connection),* New York: Boundary Books.

Pearsall, P., Schwartz, G. R. and Russek, L. S. 2002. Changes in Heart Transplant Recipients That Parallel the Personalities of Their Donors. *Journal of Near-Death Studies,* 20, 191–206.

Pedersen, S., Spindler, H., Johansen, J. B., Mortensen, P. T. and Sears, S. F. 2008. Correlates of Patient Acceptance of the Cardioverter Defibrillator: Cross-Validation of the Florida Patient Acceptance Survey in Danish Patients. *Pacing and Clinical Electrophysiology,* 31, 1168–1171.

Pelletier, D., Gallagher, R., Mitten-Lewis, S., Mckinley, S. and Squire, J. 2002. Australian Implantable Cardiac Defibrillator Recipients: Quality-of-life Issues. *International Journal of Nursing Practice,* 8, 68–74.

Penley, C., Ross, A. and Haraway, D. 1990. Cyborgs at Large: Interview with Donna Haraway. *Social Text,* 25/26, 8–23.

Persson, M. O., Persson, N. H., Ranstam, J. and Hermeren, G. 2003. Xenotransplantation Public Perceptions: Rather Cells than Organs. *Xenotransplantation,* 10, 72–79.

Piot, O., Deballon, R., Nitu, D., Marquié, C., Da Costa, A., Leclercq, C., Defaye, P. and Sadoul, N. 2015. Factors Predicting Sprint Fidelis Lead Fracture: Results at 5 Years from a French Multicentre Registry. *Archives of Cardiovascular Diseases,* 108, 220–226.

Pollock, A. 2011. The Internal Cardiac Defibrillator. In: S. Turkle (ed.), *The Inner History of Devices.* Cambridge, MA: MIT Press.

Quigley, M. and Ayihongbe, S. 2018. Everyday Cyborgs: On Integrated Persons and Integrated Goods. *Medical Law Review,* 26, 276–308.

Radcliffe, J. 2011. Hacking Medical Devices for Fun and Insulin: Breaking the Human SCADA System. https://paper.bobylive.com/Meeting_Papers/BlackHat/USA-2011/BH_US_11_Radcliffe_Hacking_Medical_Devices_WP.pdf (accessed December 2020).

Ransford, B., Clark, S. S., Kune, D. F., Fu, K. and Burleson, W. P. 2014. Design Challenges for Secure Implantable Medical Devices. In: W. Burleson and S. Carrara (eds.), *Security and Privacy for Implantable Medical Devices.* New York: Springer.

Rémy, C. 2014. 'Men Seeking Monkey-glands': The Controversial Xenotransplantations of Doctor Voronoff, 1910–30. *French History,* 28, 226–240.

Rimmer, A. 2018. Vaginal Mesh Procedures Need Compulsory Register, Says Royal College. *British Medical Journal,* 360, k586.

Rios, A., Conesa, C., Ramirez, P., Galindo, P. J., Rodriguez, J. M., Montoya, M. J. and Parrilla, P. 2005. Attitude Toward Xenotransplantation Among Residents. *Transplantation Proceedings,* 37, 4111–4116.

Robert, J. S. and Baylis, F. 2003. Crossing Species Boundaries. *American Journal of Bioethics,* 3, 1–13.

Roberts, P. 2011. Blind Attack on Wireless Insulin Pumps Could Deliver Lethal Dose. *Threatpost (blog post).* https://threatpost.com/blind-attack-wireless-insulin-pumps-could-deliver-lethal-dose-102711/75808/ (accessed December 2020).

Russo, J. E. 2011. Original Research: Deactivation of ICDs at the End Of Life: A Systematic Review of Clinical Practices and Provider and Patient Attitudes. *American Journal of Nursing,* 111, 26–35.

Sakensa, S. 1994. The Impact of Implantable Cardioverter Defibrillator Therapy on Health Care Systems. *American Heart Journal,* 127, 1193–1200.

Sanal, A. 2011. *New Organs Within Us: Transplants and the Moral Economy,* Durham and London: Duke University Press.

References

Sanner, M. A. 1998. Giving and Taking: To Whom and From Whom? People's Attitudes Toward Transplantation of Organs and Tissue from Different Sources. *Clinical Transplantation*, 12, 530–537.

Sanner, M. A. 2001a. Exchanging Spare Parts or Becoming a New Person? People's Attitudes Toward Receiving and Donating Organs. *Social Science and Medicine*, 1491–1499.

Sanner, M. A. 2001b. People's Feelings and Ideas about Receiving Transplants of Different Origins Questions of Life and Death, Identity, and Nature's Border. *Clinical Transplantation*, 15, 19–27.

Sanner, M. A. 2003. Transplant Recipients' Conceptions of Three Key Phenomena in Transplantation: The Organ Donation, the Organ Donor, and the Organ Transplant. *Clinical Transplantation*, 17, 391–400.

Sanner, M. A. 2006. People's Attitudes and Reactions to Organ Donation. *Mortality*, 11, 133–150.

Savulescu, J. and Bostrom, N. (eds.) 2009. *Human Enhancement*, Oxford: Oxford University Press.

Schraube, E. 2009. Technology as Materialized Action and Its Ambivalences. *Theory & Psychology*, 19, 296–312.

Sears, S. F. and Conti, J. B. 2003. Understanding Implantable Cardioverter Defibrillator Shocks and Storms: Medical and Psychosocial Considerations for Research and Clinical Care. *Clinical Cardiology*, 26, 107–111.

Sears, S. F., Todaro, J., Lewis, T., Sotile, W. and Conti, J. B. 1999. Examining the Psychosocial Impact of Implantable Cardioverter Defibrillators: A Literature Review. *Clinical Cardiology*, 22, 481–489.

Sharp, L. 1995. Organ Transplantation as a Transformative Experience: Anthropological Insights into the Restructuring of the Self. *Medical Anthropology Quarterly*, 9, 372.

Sharp, L. 2006. *Strange Harvest: Organ Transplants, Denatured Bodies, and the Transformed Self,* California: University of California Press.

Shelley, M. [1831] 1993. *Frankenstein or The Modern Prometheus,* Hertfordshire: Wordsworth Editions Limited.

Sheper-Hughes, N. and Lock, M. 1987. The Mindful Body: A Prolegomenon to Future Work in Medical Anthropology. *Medical Anthropology Quarterly*, 1, 6–41.

Shildrick, M. 2010. Some Reflections on the Socio-cultural and the Bioscientific Limits of Bodily Integrity. *Body & Society*, 16, 11–22.

Shildrick, M. 2014. Visceral Phenomenology: Organ Transplantation, Identity and Sexual Difference. In: L. Kall and K. Zeiler (eds.), *Feminist Phenomenology and Medicine*, New York: Suny Press.

Shildrick, M. 2015. Staying Alive: Affect, Identity and Anxiety in Organ Transplantation. *Body & Society*, 21, 20–41.

Shildrick, M., Mckeever, P., Abbey, S., Poole, J. and Ross, H. 2009. Troubling Dimensions of Heart Transplantation. *Medical Humanities*, 35, 35–38.

Shilling, C. 2001. Embodiment, Experience and Theory: In Defence of the Sociological Tradition. *Sociological Review*, 49, 328–344.

Shilling, C. and Mellor, P. 1996. Embodiment, Structuration Theory and Modernity: Mind/Body Dualism and the Repression of Sensuality. *Body and Society*, 2, 1–15.

Shpiner, D. S., Di Luca, D. G., Cajigas, I., Diaz, J. S., Margolesky, J., Moore, H., Levin, B. E., Singer, C., Jagid, J. and Luca, C. C. 2019. Gender Disparities in Deep Brain Stimulation for Parkinson's Disease. *Neuromodulation: Technology at the Neural Interface*, 22, 484–488.

Simmons, R., Klein, M. and Simmons, R. (eds.) 1987. *Gift of Life: The Effect of Organ Transplantation on Individual, Family and Societal Dynamics*, Oxford: Transaction Books.

Singer, P. 1994. *Re-Thinking Life and Death: The Collapse of Our Traditional Ethics*, Oxford: Oxford University Press.

Slatman, J. and Widdershoven, G. 2010. Hand Transplants and Bodily Integrity. *Body & Society*, 16, 69–92.

Smith, G. J. D. 2016. Surveillance, Data and Embodiment: On the Work of Being Watched. *Body & Society*, 22(2), 108–139.

Sobchack, V. 2010. Living a 'Phantom Limb': On the Phenomenology of Bodily Integrity. *Body & Society*, 16, 51–67.

Spindler, H., Johansen, J. B., Andersen, K., Mortensen, P. and Pedersen, S. S. 2009. Gender Differences in Anxiety and Concerns about the Cardioverter Defibrillator. *PACE – Pacing and Clinical Electrophysiology*, 32, 614–621.

Stadlbauer, V., Stiegler, P., Müller, S., Schweiger, M., Sereingg, M., Tscheliessnigg, K. H. and Freidl, W. 2011. Attitude toward Xenotransplantation of Patients Prior and After Human Organ Transplantation. *Clinical Transplantation*, 25, 495–503.

Standing, H. C., Rapley, T., Macgowan, G. A. and Exley, C. 2017. 'Being' a Ventricular Assist Device Recipient: A Liminal Existence. *Social Science & Medicine*, 190, 141–148.

Starrenburg, A., Pedersen, S., Van Den Broek, K., Kraaier, K., Scholten, M. and Van Der Palen, J. 2014. Gender Differences in Psychological Distress and Quality of Life in Patients with an ICD 1-year Postimplant. *PACE – Pacing and Clinical Electrophysiology*, 37, 843–852.

Starzl, T. E., Demetris, A. J., Trucco, M., Murase, N., Ricordi, C., Ildstad, S., Ramos, H., Todo, S., Tzakis, A., Fung, J. J., Nalesnik, M., Zeevi, A., Rudert, W. A. and Kocova, M. 1993. Cell Migration and Chimerism After Whole-organ Transplantation: The Basis of Graft Acceptance. *Hepatology (Baltimore, Md.)*, 17, 1127–1152.

Steinke, E. E., Gill-Hopple, K., Valdez, D. and Wooster, M. 2005. Sexual Concerns and Educational Needs After an Implantable Cardioverter Defibrillator. *Heart & Lung*, 34, 299–308.

Stinson, M. and Buckley, G. (eds.) 2013. *New Beginnings: Acquiring and Living with a Cochlear Implant*, Rochester: RIT Press.

Sulik, G. A. 2009. Managing Biomedical Uncertainty: The Technoscientific Illness Identity. *Sociology of Health & Illness*, 31, 1059–1076.

Sulik, G. A. 2011. 'Our Diagnoses, Our Selves': The Rise of the Technoscientific Illness Identity. *Sociology Compass*, 5, 463–477.

Swierstra, T., Van Est, R. and Boenink, M. 2009. Taking Care of the Symbolic Order. How Converging Technologies Challenge our Concepts. *Nanoethics,* doi: 10.1007/s11569–009–0080–0.

Sylvia, C. and Novack, W. 1997. *A Change Of Heart; The Extraordinary Story of a Man's Heart in a Woman's Body*, Little Brown: London.

Tagney, J., James, J. E. and Albarran, J. W. 2003. Exploring the Patient's Experiences of Learning to Live with an Implantable Cardioverter Defibrillator (ICD) from One UK Centre: A Qualitative Study. *European Journal of Cardiovascular Nursing*, 2, 195–203.

Taylor-Alexander, S. 2004. *On Face Transplantation: Life and Ethics in Experimental Biomedicine*, Palgrave Pivot Macmillan: London.

Tchou, P., Piasecki, E., Gutman, M., Jazayeri, M., Axtell, K. and Akhtar, M. 1989. Psychological Support and Psychiatric Management of Patients with Automatic Implantable Cardioverter Defribillators. *International Journal of Psychiatry Medicine*, 1989, 393–407.

Teran-Escandon, D., Teran-Ortiz, L., Ormsby-Jenkins, C., Evia-Viscarra, M. L., White, D. J. G. and Valdes-Gonzalez-Salas, R. 2005. Psychosocial Aspects of Xenotransplantation: Survey in Adolescent Recipients of Porcine Islet Cells. *Transplantation Proceedings*, 37, 521–524.

Theodorakopoulou, E., Meghji, S., Pafitanis, G. and Mason, K. A. 2017. A Review of the World's Published Face Transplant Cases: Ethical Perspectives. *Scars, Burns & Healing*, 3, 2059513117694402.

Timmermans, S. and Berg, M. 2003. The Practice of Medical Technology. *Sociology of Health & Illness*, 25, 97–114.

Turkle, S. (ed.) 2011. *The Inner History of Devices*, Cambridge, MA: Massachusetts Institute of Technology.

Turner, B. 1992. *Regulating Bodies: Essays in Medical Sociology*, London, Routledge.

Turner, B. S. 2008. *The Body and Society: Exploration in Social Theory*, London: Sage.

Valente, J. M. 2011. Cyborgization: Deaf Education for Young Children in the Cochlear Implantation Era. *Qualitative Inquiry*, 17, 639–652.

Van Den Broek, K. C., Nyklíček, I., Van Der Voort, P. H., Alings, M., Meijer, A. and Denollet, J. 2009. Risk of Ventricular Arrhythmia After Implantable Defibrillator Treatment in Anxious Type D Patients. *Journal of the American College of Cardiology,* 54, 531–537.

Van Den Eede, Y. 2015. Where Is the Human? Beyond the Enhancement Debate. *Science, Technology & Human Values,* 40, 149–162.

Varela, F. 2001. Intimate Distances: Fragments for a Phenomenology of Organ Transplantation. *Journal of Consciousness Studies,* 8, 259–271.

Vermeulen, N., Haddow, G., Seymour, T., Faulkner-Jones, A. and Shu, W. 2017. 3D Bioprint Me: A Socioethical View of Bioprinting Human Organs and Tissues. *Journal of Medical Ethics,* 43(8), 618–624.

Vidal, F. 2009. Brainhood, Anthropological Figure of Modernity. *History of the Human Sciences,* 22, 5–36.

Vriesendorp, P. A., Schinkel, A. F. L., Cleemput, J. V., Willems, R., Jordaens, L. J. L., Theuns, D. A. M. J., Van Slegtenhorst, M. A., De Ravel, T. J., Ten Cate, F. J. and Michels, M. 2013. Implantable Cardioverter-defibrillators in Hypertrophic Cardiomyopathy: Patient Outcomes, Rate of Appropriate and Inappropriate Interventions, and Complications. *American Heart Journal,* 166, 496–502.

Warwick, K. 2003. Cyborg Morals, Cyborg Values, Cyborg Ethics. *Ethics Information and Technology,* 5, 131–137.

Warwick, K. 2004. *I, Cyborg,* Illinois: University of Illinois Press (Reprint edition).

Warwick, K. 2008. Prosthetics: A User Guide for Posthumans. *The American Journal of Psychology,* 121, 161–166.

Warwick, K., Gasson, M., Hutt, B., Goodhew, I., Kyberd, P., Andrews, B., Teddy, P. and Shad, A. 2003. The Application of Implant Technology in Cybernetic Systems. *Archives of Neurology,* 60, 1369–1373.

Waskul, D. and Vannini, P. 2006. *Body/Embodiment: Symbolic Interaction and the Sociology of the Body,* Aldershot: Ashgate.

Waskul, D. D. and Riet, P. V. D. 2002. The Abject Embodiment of Cancer Patients: Dignity, Selfhood, and the Grotesque Body. *Symbolic Interaction,* 25, 487–513.

Weiss, G. 1999. *Body Images: Embodiment as Intercorporeality,* London and New York: Routledge.

Welin, S. and Sandrin, M. S. 2006. Some Ethical Problems in Xenotransplant ation: Introductory Remarks at Ethics Workshop. *Xenotransplantation,* 13, 500–501.

Wenger, N. K. 2004. You've Come a Long Way, Baby: Cardiovascular Health and Disease in Women: Problems and Prospects. *Circulation,* 109, 558–560.

Whang, W., Albert, C. M., Sears jr, S. F., Lampert, R., Conti, J. B., Wang, P. J., Singh, J. P., Ruskin, J. N., Muller, J. E. and Mittleman, M. A. 2005. Depression as a Predictor for Appropriate Shocks Among Patients with Implantable Cardioverter-defibrillators : Results from the Triggers of Ventricular Arrhythmias (TOVA) Study. *Journal of the American College of Cardiology*, 45, 1090–1095.

White, M. M. 2002. Psychosocial Impact of the Implantable Cardioverter Defibrillator: Nursing Implications. *Journal of Cardiovascular Nursing*, 16, 53–61.

Wiener, N. 1961. *Cybernetics or Control and Communication in the Animal and the Machine*, Cambridge, MA: MIT Press.

Williams, S. J. 1997. Modern Medicine and the 'Uncertain Body': From Corporeality to Hyperreality? *Social Science and Medicine*, 45, 1041–1049.

Williams, M. and Penman, D. 2014. *Mindfulness: A Practical Guide to Finding Peace in a Frantic World*, London: Piatkus.

Winner, L. 1993. Upon Opening the Black Box and Finding it Empty: Social Constructivism and the Philosophy of Technology. *Science, Technology & Human Values*, 18, 362–378.

Wise, J. 2016. Permanent Mesh Has 'Limited Utility' for Vaginal Prolapse Repair, Review Finds. *British Medical Journal*, 352, i822.

Wise, J. 2017. NICE to Ban Mesh for Vaginal Wall Prolapse. *British Medical Journal*, 359, j5523.

Withell, B. 2006. Patient Consent and Implantable Cardioverter Defibrillators: Some Palliative Care Implications. *International Journal of Palliative Nursing*, 12, 470–475.

Yarnoz, M. J. and Curtis, A. B. 2006. Sex-based Differences in Cardiac Resynchronization Therapy and Implantable Cardioverter Defibrillator Therapies: Effectiveness and Use. *Cardiology in Review*, 14, 292–298.

Yuhas, J., Mattocks, K., Gravelin, L., Remetz, M., Foley, J., Fazio, R. and Lampert, R. 2012. Patients' Attitudes and Perceptions of Implantable Cardioverter-defibrillators. *Pacing and Clinical Electrophysiology*, 35, 1179–1187.

Index

EU authorised representative for GPSR:
Easy Access System Europe, Mustamäe tee 50,
10621 Tallinn, Estonia
gpsr.requests@easproject.com